The Tooth, the Whole Tooth and Nothing but the Tooth!

Dr Sarita Subramaniam, BDS, graduated from the Government Dental College and Hospital, Mumbai. She has been managing her private dental practice in Mumbai for the last twenty years and focuses on endodontics, restorative and prosthetic dentistry. She loves working with children and her little patients vouch for her gentle hands. She's also a passionate writer, animal activist and wildlife lover, and is presently completing a book on birdwatching! She extends her expertise in dentistry to rendering dental treatment to dogs and cats, too, at a veterinary facility in Mumbai.

Dr P.V. Subramaniam, MDS, completed his education as a periodontist from the Nair Hospital Dental College, Mumbai. He was closely associated with academics for over fifteen years, and last held the post of a professor and the head of the Department of Periodontics at the MGM Dental College and Hospital, Navi Mumbai. He has also been a consultant in private practice since 1995 and focuses on periodontics, minor oral surgery, endodontics and implantology. He has published a book on English humour and is an accomplished wildlife photographer. He joins his wife, Sarita in rendering dental care to suffering animals.

Both authors conduct free dental camps for those in remote locations such as forest guards and villagers staying around forests. They are also involved with charitable work for marginalized communities to whom they distribute solar lamps and daily necessities. They work for the welfare of stray dogs in Mumbai, and care for over twenty-five of them by ensuring that they are fed daily and vaccinated against disease. They also manage an organic farm at Karjat, near Mumbai, where they have demonstrated the virtues of avoiding chemical fertilizers and pesticides. They live in Mumbai with a cat and three dogs.

The Tooth, the Whole Tooth and Nothing but the Tooth!

A complete guide to dental care

Dr Sarita Subramaniam
Dr P.V. Subramaniam

Illustrated by Anita Sundareswaran

RUPA

To our parents

Published by
Rupa Publications India Pvt. Ltd 2015
7/16, Ansari Road, Daryaganj
New Delhi 110002

Sales Centres:

Allahabad Bengaluru Chennai
Hyderabad Jaipur Kathmandu
Kolkata Mumbai

While every effort has been made to verify the authenticity of the
information contained in this book, it is not intended as a substitute for
medical consultation with a physician. The publisher and the author are in no
way liable for the use of the information contained in this book

ISBN 978-81-2913-719-7

First impression 2015

10 9 8 7 6 5 4 3 2 1

The moral right of the author has been asserted.

This edition is for sale in the Indian Subcontinent only.

Contents

Introduction:
A Nibble of This Book

The lives of most people follow a reasonably steady course, filled largely with the prosaic and the mundane. Adventure, adrenaline, fear, thrills—these are few and far between. But life's humdrum journey changes rapidly when a dreaded event approaches: *the dental appointment!* One goes weak-kneed, the boldest quiver, and given a choice—wild horses couldn't drag one into the dentist's chamber.

Knowledge dispels the darkness of ignorance, and is the greatest weapon to quell irrational fears. This book, therefore, squarely addresses—at the outset—the problem of 'dental' anxiety, and once the jangled nerves have calmed down, seeks to gently educate the reader about the truly *wonderful* modern science of dentistry. Let's take a whistle-stop tour of this tome!

The book first gives you a peek into the structure and functions of teeth. It affirms their vital importance, and the crucial need to hold on to them for the rest of our dear lives.

Tooth decay has been the bane of mankind from the time we came down from the trees and started eating junk! A large section of this book is, therefore, devoted to understanding dental cavities: how they occur, why they cause toothache, their treatment and prevention.

Sensitive teeth can be a real pain! What are the options for dealing with this? Are desensitizing toothpastes effective? Do mouthwashes help? Can the dentist treat this affliction?

A sensitive look at this irksome issue is to be found in the pages of this book.

But it's not just teeth—our gums, too, need attention, and gum disease is one of the most common conditions found in any population, married to bad breath and loose teeth. This syndrome does not distinguish between kings or paupers. Apart from causing damage to the teeth, it has now been proven to have dark links to cardiovascular disease.

Then there's bad breath—known to deprive people of close encounters! It is, therefore, important to know this adversary—its symptoms, its progression, how to prevent it, and the various options available for its treatment.

Along the way, we offer advice. A case in point—don't gnash your teeth! Believe it or not, bruxism (and that's its name!) is a real problem—it wears away the teeth, and the jaw joint, and leaves one weary! Here, we take a close look at this peculiar habit, which is far more rampant than estimated.

We also consider two special sets of people—kids and expectant moms—and tackle all the buzzwords that concern them: nursing, teething, milk teeth, fluoride! Their unique dental problems, and the solutions, are addressed in simple language, so that the foundation for dental health can be laid early.

We believe that charity—and dental care—both begin at home! All that one wants to know about toothbrushing, flossing and mouthwashes are explained in the context of home care, the greatest weapon in the war against dental maladies.

It's not just armies that march on their stomachs—even our teeth do! Good nutrition is vital to ensure that your pearlies glow white and bite right.

★

Yes, we are well aware that our reputation precedes us. Dentists are most feared for drilling and filling. But hey, we are here to dispel those myths! Have your fill of information on the latest *pain-free* techniques and materials for these procedures.

Root canal treatments are lifesaving procedures for teeth. They have become painless (there's the word again!), fast and even more effective than before. Take a tour of the insides of the tooth to marvel at this treatment.

While dentists today go to great lengths to preserve our teeth, those beyond redemption fall prey to the forceps. An overview of tooth extractions is provided, to understand why and which teeth need to be removed, and what to expect if one must undergo the procedure. Several other questions about tooth removal—which prey on the mind—are also answered. Wisely, surgical extractions, especially of wisdom teeth, are also dealt with.

Teeth are lost due to several reasons, and replacing them is of vital importance. From its humble beginnings in the form of removable dentures, this science of prosthetic dentistry has come a long way. The plethora of contemporary options, from high-end removable dentures to bridges and dental implants, are discussed. Modern dentistry does not believe in an eye for an eye, but certainly in a tooth for a tooth!

Any mention of orthodontic treatment, and people 'brace' themselves for the shocking bill! However, as expensive as it is, there is no alternative to putting misaligned teeth in order: the face structure improves, speech clears, the ability to chew eases, and confidence soars.

Most dental treatments are performed with an eye firmly fixed on maintaining aesthetics: gum treatments, fillings and tooth replacements. However, cosmetic dentistry specifically focuses on giving people a billion-dollar smile, at a smaller cost though! This modern aspect of dentistry has become hugely popular, and most people are now aware of tooth bleaching, laminates, etc. Various techniques available today—to convert beastly teeth into beauties—are discussed too.

★

Truth be told, a visit to the dental clinic need not be only about teeth. The mouth is a mirror of the body, and dentists can often diagnose the presence of other diseases or conditions by examining the oral cavity. Diabetes, hormonal imbalances, emotional stress, vitamin deficiencies, HIV, leukaemia, oral cancer—little escapes the dentist's lens.

And finally, some questions which are rarely answered: What are your expectations from your dentist? Can they be addressed? What makes a good dental office/clinic? Do you really need to rob a bank to afford dental care? This book tries to venture into these uncharted territories.

So, between the covers, welcome to a world where we promise to tell the tooth, the whole tooth, and nothing but the tooth!

Chapter 1

Dental Anxiety:
Find Your Peace

Calm. Soothing. Solace. Tranquil. Relaxed.
These are not words people imagine when referring to dental treatment. Most folks develop cold feet at the very mention of visiting the dentist, who is often the favourite target of satirists and stand-up comedians. Each of us knows of at least one dentist joke, but guess who has the last laugh, though—teeth or no teeth, everyone needs the dentist!

Early Fears: Doctors and Demons

In today's times, dentists are specialists who not only treat the mouth and teeth, but also aid greatly in improving one's persona and self-esteem. Modern equipment, better materials and the widespread use of effective local anaesthesia, have helped dentists render most dental procedures painless.

Why are dentists, then, still the most dreaded amongst doctors? Fear of pain during treatment remains quite deep-rooted in most people. This

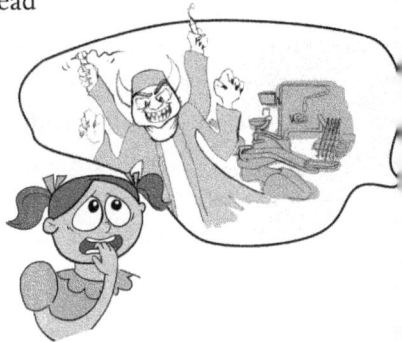

stems from the rather unpleasant history of the evolution of dentistry as a profession. In fact, in the olden days, it was barbers who doubled up to provide dental treatment, including tooth extractions!

Terror, anxiety and apprehension are common feelings strongly associated with a dental appointment. There are a handful of reasons for this.

A lot has to do with our childhood conditioning, of the societal imagery of the dentist as a forceps-wielding monster! If parents are scared to go to their dentist, then their apprehensions would be passed on to their children, albeit non-verbally. Parents often instil the fear of the dentist's 'injection' into the child's mind, when the poor kid shies away from brushing her teeth. Worse still, many children are subjected to a common threat by parents: 'Brush your teeth, or else the dentist will pull them out!'

Imagine a groggy child, visualizing an ogre in a white coat next to a 'sleeping' chair, brandishing a pair of forceps menacingly in a cold room bathed in white light...shiver, shiver! Therefore, when children are taken to the dental clinic for the first time, they are carrying a mountain of phobia with them.

For some, the fear of dentistry may be due to a direct association with an unpleasant dental episode in which they suffered much pain and trauma.

Many of us, though, develop this fear through hearsay! Even without having had any personal experience, we imagine the worst! There are indeed countless horror stories of how others suffered—we imagine ourselves in these situations, and get wound up!

The media also plays a role in propagating similar stereotypical stories. A number of films have portrayed dentists in a negative light, and these visual images can leave a lasting impression. A highly acclaimed movie from 1976 (*The Marathon Man*) has the antagonist torturing his victims by drilling their teeth without anaesthesia. Aargh!

We also tend to transfer memories from near-similar environments to the dental situation, making them the basis for our phobia. For example, if you have had a bad incident in a hospital setting, the sights, smells and sounds of a dental clinic may trigger that residual fear.

You may also believe that the dentist is unstoppable during a procedure! You imagine that you have no control when lying in the dental chair, and that the dentist will continue, unabated, even if you feel pain.

Is it surprising, then, that we nurture these irrational fears, deeply embedded in the recesses of our brain? The dread of pain is a deep, primitive instinct, leading us to avoid situations with the potential to inflict it. Undoubtedly, this is the primary reason for the fear of dental treatment.

Tender Tooth Care: No Pain, All Gain

Fortunately, in today's dental clinic, the emphasis is on making *all* treatment painless! Vast improvements have taken place over the years regarding local anaesthetic drugs, which totally banish pain!

Currently, we have drugs that are potent, long acting, and extremely safe. Even the method of injecting them has become refined—disposable, factory-sharpened needles are barely felt when entering the body, and numbness follows rapidly thereafter. Most dentists are also, now, careful to administer the injection ultra-slowly, so that the pressure of the liquid penetrating the tissues is minimized.

Dentists, nowadays, prefer using local anaesthesia for *most* procedures, including fillings, and this keeps all forms of treatment pain-free! Since there is a wide safety margin in present-day local anaesthetics, dentists do not hesitate to give additional doses in case of any hurt during the process. In fact, most of them prime their patients to indicate their discomfort if any, during a procedure, using a predetermined signal. The dentist will stop the procedure immediately, and administer a little more of the anaesthetic if needed. Thus, you *do* remain in total control of the situation!

The numbness on account of the local anaesthesia can be a bit of an impediment—the lips, cheek and tongue feel lifeless, causing temporary speech impairment, drooling, inadvertent injury, etc. A new drug called OraVerse™ (containing phentolamine) injected into the area, quickly reverses this numbness, allowing you to go about your activities without any inconvenience.

The latest development is the computer-controlled injecting system (example: The Wand™), which address many of the issues regarding a routine injection. First, it doesn't look like a syringe; it is more like a ballpoint pen, and is held like one. Second, a device controls the speed of the injection, letting the anaesthetic solution move in very slowly. It uses super fine needles, and can be restricted to numbing just the tooth in question. This means no loss of sensation in the lips, cheek and tongue!

Overcoming Phobia: Conquering the Senses

Apart from the fear of pain, there are diverse triggers for anxiety in a dental setting, which contribute to the associated phobia. For one, a dental clinic can surely look intimidating!

The dental chair is surrounded by many arms, which hold various types of equipment. A powerful light shines into your eyes while the dentist attends to your teeth, making you feel like a suspect under interrogation.

Worse, lots of scary-looking instruments are passed around and used within the mouth. Some feel cold and uncomfortable to the touch. Most people flinch when the dental drill starts off, which *can* get quite noisy! The smell of disinfectants could also spark recollections of a hospital setting, which many of us abhor.

Therefore, there is a *multi-sensory* reaction to the elements in a dental office, all of which add to the anxiety level.

Dental phobia, or anxiety, is widely recognized *and* acknowledged as a serious hurdle to delivering good dental care. Dentists, generally, go the extra mile when it comes to keeping you comfortable, and in a positive frame of mind. They spend more time in explaining treatment procedures and expected outcomes, so that there are no surprises—uncertainty is a source of stress! Many misconceptions can be cleared up, and when you understand the nature of the processes, they are often not as torturous as you imagined!

The initial meeting is often scheduled in a separate area, and not the operatory, so as to minimize environmental stress. Dentists tend to begin treatment with minor, easy-going procedures rather than plunge into a complicated one at the outset. This allows a gradual easing into the interventions, a soft launch, so to speak.

The décor and ambience of a dental clinic can go a long way in soothing the nerves! Soft lighting and pastel shades are being increasingly deployed to soften the harshness of a surgical environment; warm tones can help overcome the fear of the aseptic, tiled look. For those who are very anxious, eye masks (similar to those found in aircrafts) can keep the unnerving sights away—please ask your dentist for one!

Techno-savvy dentists offer DVD glasses—slip them on, and choose your favourite movie or TV programme to enjoy while the dentist fixes your teeth! Most clinics now play piped music to lighten the atmosphere.

Dental drills operate with high-pressure compressed air, and this results in a high-pitched whine. Modern versions have managed to keep the pitch much lower with improved designs. Electrically-operated drills have also been developed to further minimize the sound. Noise-cancelling headphones can help those who want to block out the racket of drilling and other dental machinery.

Newer air-abrasion techniques use a fine stream of pressurized abrasive powders to clean out tooth decay without drills. This translates into an almost soundless affair, and is handy for treating small cavities. Lasers are also being employed to replace drilling in some situations; these, too, are noiseless, and often need no anaesthesia.

Dental clinics are like mini operation theatres. They need a high standard of cleanliness, for which powerful disinfectants are used. These emit a 'hospital' smell, which can evoke unpleasant associations. Several clinics choose disinfectants that are almost odourless, or have added fragrances to mask any residual smell. Another recourse is to place fragrance diffusers and aromatherapy oils to set a relaxed tone at the dental office.

A new application is currently claiming good results in the management of dental phobia. The system called NuCalm™, has four different components to tackle various anxiety inducers. Patients are first asked to chew tablets containing GABA (gamma-aminobutyric acid), a chemical which is normally present in the brain and calms the nerves. It is not a prescription drug; it is sold as a supplement. Next, small patches, called micro-current stimulators, are placed behind their ears and hooked up to a device, which transmits tiny electrical currents to soothe the brain waves. Headphones that play special acoustic software to blank out noises are clamped to the ears. Finally, dark glasses are slipped on, to block out visual stimuli. The system claims to transport patients into a relaxed, pre-sleep stage, where there is no feeling of apprehension.

In rare instances, the above measures might still not serve to allay deep-rooted anxiety. To reduce the tension, dentists may then recommend medication, such as Alprazolam, to be taken a few hours prior to the treatment. Extremely nervous patients would need the last-resort options—they'd need to be put under sedation, or even general anaesthesia.

Dental clinics and offices have been highly responsive to the ubiquitous nature of dental anxiety. The focus is not only on relieving the apprehension, but also on making the dental experience something that you actually look forward to!

Myths and Misconceptions: Getting Your Sums Right

As if there weren't enough reasons to provoke fear, there are innumerable myths and misconceptions associated with teeth and dentists, adding fuel to the fire! Often, it is an uphill task for the dentist to deal with unscientific, preconceived ideas. They have to then help their patients with not just treating the disease, but also in dispelling these irrational notions surrounding dental treatment.

Myth: Removal of Upper Teeth Can Cause Blindness or Brain Damage

The truth is that while the upper and lower teeth do have nerve endings which originate in the brain, extracting them doesn't even remotely lead to brain damage... the perpetrator of this myth perhaps suffered from it! Similarly, one doesn't become blind by extracting the upper teeth, just because of their proximity to the eyes!

Misconception: Don't Brush Your Teeth When You Have Bleeding Gums

Gums bleed as a result of inflammation caused by germs adhering to the teeth. If you discontinue oral hygiene practices, the bleeding will worsen! Keep brushing and flossing, and see your dentist soon.

Myth: Teeth Become Loose with Frequent Cleaning at the Dentist's

People assume that since they clean their teeth regularly at home, there is no need for a routine dental checkup. Teeth, however, are not user-friendly when it comes to maintenance. While home care is mandatory, teeth need professional cleaning (called *scaling*) at regular intervals to ensure freedom from tartar deposition.

In the early days, scaling was performed by a manual scraping technique, which resulted in the operator applying force on the teeth. Contemporary equipments ensure that the process doesn't even scratch them!

Teeth already loosened by gum disease, but held together by a thick layer of tartar deposits, could feel suddenly loose after scaling. In these instances, the procedure only exposes the true state of the tooth's weakness—it doesn't cause the looseness!

In fact, scaling also offers a good opportunity to get each tooth examined closely, and detect emerging problems. Needless to say, untreated tartar deposition eventually leads to gum disease and tooth loss... the mouth does get totally cleaned out!

Misconception: 'No Toothache' Means 'No Dental Problem'

A very common statement reverberating in the dental clinic is: 'But Doctor, I don't have any problem, as I have no pain!'

It is a tough myth to dispel, as lack of pain is often considered a sign of good health. It is, however, imperative to understand that pain is, unfortunately, a very poor indicator of one's health, especially oral. Teeth vary widely in their response to disease or injury: for example, some shallow cavities may hurt like hell, while deeper ones may be totally painless; some teeth decay so completely that their entire structure collapses, but the residual roots remain pain-free!

Myth: Home Remedies Are Effective in Relieving Toothache

When teeth hurt, the first response is to lean towards home remedies. Clove oil is often massaged on painful, decaying teeth. While the active ingredient of the oil, eugenol, helps in soothing toothache, cloves and clove oil are actually a severe irritant to the gums, and should be totally avoided. Dentists see many cases of raw, burning gums caused by the application of clove oil.

Similarly, people use tobacco or even nail polish (absurd as it may sound) on painful teeth, causing much damage. Some feel that a crushed aspirin tablet applied to the tooth will relieve the pain. Actually, aspirin causes severe chemical burns to the gums, aggravating the already agonizing toothache.

It is indeed sad that the dentist is usually consulted long

after such detrimental remedies have been tried, failed and have made matters worse.

Misconception: You Can Afford to Lose Teeth

The notion that teeth are dispensable is often a major cause for avoiding dental treatment. 'If my tooth goes bad, I'll get it knocked off!'—dentists hear this statement at least once every day in their practice!

It is often challenging to convince people to hold on to their natural teeth.

Teeth function as a unit, and the loss of some teeth affects the performance and life of those that remain. Missing teeth set up a vicious cycle, accelerating the vulnerability of the others.

Myth: Teeth Will Fall Off Anyway When You Get Old

An octogenarian doesn't expect her little toe to fall off due to age! Surely, she will not be gutsy enough to remove her aging spleen just because she turned eighty...not really!

Similarly, teeth are supposed to last a lifetime! Like any other body part that undergoes wear and tear, they are also subject to normal attrition—but with proper care, your teeth can remain healthy and functional for life!

Misconception: Milk Teeth Don't Need Treatment and Are Going to Fall Off Anyway

Milk teeth are crucial for kids! They help to perform many functions, including chewing, speech, and supporting a pleasant face structure. These teeth also reserve the space for the permanent teeth that will replace them later.

Cavities in milk teeth result in pain and discomfort, and neglecting them can lead to their premature loss. Dentists advise extraction only if it the tooth cannot be saved, or if it is very close to its scheduled time of natural shedding.

Myth: Getting Your Tooth Pulled Out Is Painful

Teeth are never extracted without first administering shots of local anaesthesia—in fact, the dentist will check for total and profound numbness before commencing the operation. Some sensation of pressure is felt when a firm tooth is removed, but there is *no* pain!

Potent local anaesthetics, proper sterilization of instruments, and scientific treatment methods have ensured that the dreaded 'tooth extraction' is uneventful in the modern dental clinic. More often than not, unless absolutely necessary, the dentist avoids prescribing antibiotics, and the patient can manage with simple painkillers after the procedure.

Notwithstanding all these myths, excuses and impediments, when people finally land up at the clinic, they come to realize that the dentist is not—after all—the demon they had imagined! Present-day practitioners are sensitive to the need for assuaging the fear and apprehensions of their patients. The happy result is that, even the most fretful 'victim' leaves the dental clinic with a broad smile!

Chapter 2

A Dental Lesson:
Let's Peek Inside the Mouth

To understand the importance of teeth, it would be helpful to learn a bit about their role and their structure.

The Function of Teeth: The Role of a Lifetime

The mouth is the entrance to the gastrointestinal tract, the digestive system of the body. Everything we consume has to pass this hallowed portal before it reaches the stomach.

The primary function of teeth is to chew food, also called mastication. They break down the morsels, mechanically, into smaller particles; it is only after their shearing, pounding, gnashing and mashing that the food passes through the oesophagus or food pipe.

Saliva, secreted by the salivary glands, is the teeth's collaborator in aiding ingestion, by softening the food particles into a paste. Predominately water-based, it is released as the teeth begin their job. Often, greed can also cause our mouth to water, or 'salivate' when we see or smell food!

From the mouth, food goes into the oesophagus, which carries it to the stomach and intestines. Here, the broken-down food particles, processed by the teeth and saliva, can be easily digested with the help of chemicals, like acids and enzymes.

An apt analogy for the functioning of teeth is the scraping and grating of a coconut before placing it in a food processor because obviously, the processor cannot handle large bulky pieces. It will give up, or even become dysfunctional, trying to work around those unmanageable chunks. Similarly, teeth, by breaking food into smaller pieces, help in protecting the rest of the digestive organs from over-working.

Yes, it's true that teeth have several other roles to play as well: they help us in our speech, support our face structure, preserve the strength of our jawbones, make us smile better, and enhance our looks!

The Life Expectancy of Teeth: Set Forever

Unlike sharks, which have an unlimited number of teeth, we humans have a finite number of two sets—the milk teeth and the permanent teeth.

Children have twenty milk teeth, ten in each jaw, which start appearing at around six months of age. By the age of two, the eruption of milk teeth is usually complete.

Milk teeth are essential! They are crucial for children's growth, as they help in chewing properly, ensuring that the correct and nutritious food is consumed. Were it not for teeth, children would end up gulping their food whole.

The milk teeth also give shape to the jaw and face. Besides, these teeth reserve the space for the permanent ones, which are waiting in the wings, and also guide them to emerge in the right direction, so that they are well-aligned.

The thirty-two permanent teeth start breaking out at the age of six, and continue to merrily co-exist with the milk teeth for a few years. The last to appear are the wisdom teeth, so named as they surface around the age of eighteen, when one is assumed to have become wise!

Naming Those Teeth: Horses for Courses

As mammals, we have heterodont teeth—that is, teeth with different shapes, unlike our reptilian predecessors. Humans have four types of teeth, each with a different task: incisors, canines, molars and premolars. Though the first three are found in both, the milk (deciduous) and the permanent sets, the premolars are present only in the latter.

The four incisors in each jaw help in cutting or tearing-off food. Unlike the tusks of an elephant, which are in fact long, conical and pointed incisors, ours are squarish, with a flat edge.

Types of Teeth

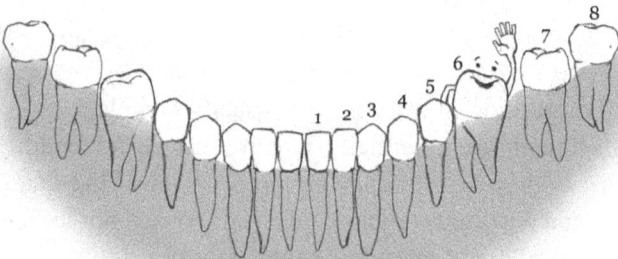

1. Central Incisor
2. Lateral Incisor
3. Canine
4. First premolar
5. Second Premolar
6. First Molar
7. Second Molar
8. Third molar (Wisdom Tooth)

The two canines in each jaw are much smaller than the ones found in the four-legged canine—man's best friend, the dog! Our strongest front teeth, canines are long, with a pointed shape like a cusp, giving significant support to the corners of the mouth. Much like that of the dog's, they tear, shear and cut, aiding the incisors in their duty.

The bulk of mastication, or chewing and grinding of sheared food, is done by the molars, usually four to six in each jaw within the permanent set of teeth. Designed to last a lifetime, these bulky teeth, or grinders, have several cusps that aid in completely pounding the food. They work like a millstone.

Premolars, four in each jaw, make an appearance only in the permanent set. Each of them has two cusps, and they assist the doughty molars in the arduous task of mastication.

A question that nags most parents is, 'Will the teeth grow bigger after they erupt fully?' Unlike rodents, our teeth don't continue to grow. The size of the jaw increases when a child grows, but the size of the human tooth remains the same from the time it comes out .

Timetables: Keeping Pace

Teeth have fixed schedules of arrival. Milk teeth exfoliate or fall when they are ready to depart to the land of the tooth fairy, at the assigned age. Dentists extract them if they have overstayed their welcome and are coming in the way of the permanent teeth. (Refer to the image: 'Milk Teeth Timetable'.)

The Crown and the Root: Getting Physical

The visible part of the tooth is just the tip of the proverbial

Milk Teeth Timetable

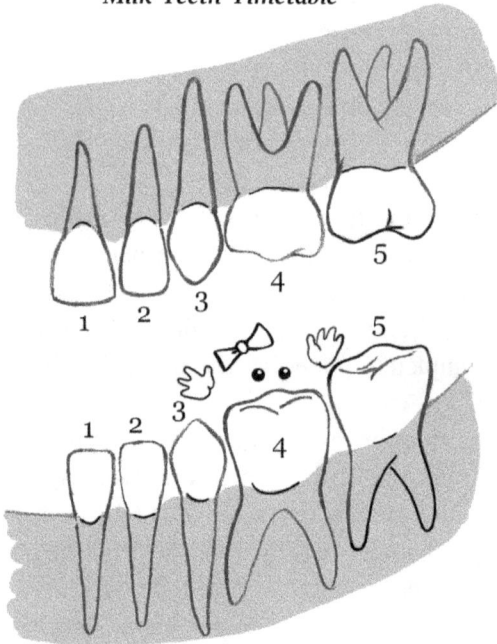

No:	Tooth	In	Out
UPPER			
1	Central Incisor	8-12 months	6-7 years
2	Lateral Incisor	9-13 months	7-8 years
3	Canine	16-22 months	10-12 years
4	First Molar	13-19 months	9-11 years
5	Second Molar	22-33 months	10-12 years
LOWER			
1	Central Incisor	6-10 months	6-7 years
2	Lateral Incisor	10-16 months	7-8 years
3	Canine	17-23 months	9-12 years
4	First Molar	14-18 months	9-11 years
5	Second Molar	23-31 months	10-12 years

iceberg! Called the 'crown', its shape varies across the incisors, canines, premolars and molars.

The submerged part of the tooth, which anchors it to the jawbone, is called the root. Incisors and canines have single roots, with the canine having the longest root of them all!

The molars and premolars have to withstand the extreme force generated by jaw muscles during the grinding of food. Premolars may have one or two roots each, lower molars usually have two, while the upper molars have three!

The Enamel and the Pulp: What's in the Box?

Teeth are constructed in layers, the outermost known as enamel. Translucent and glassy, it is extremely hardy, and resistant to damage by the different types of foodstuffs that

Parts of the Tooth

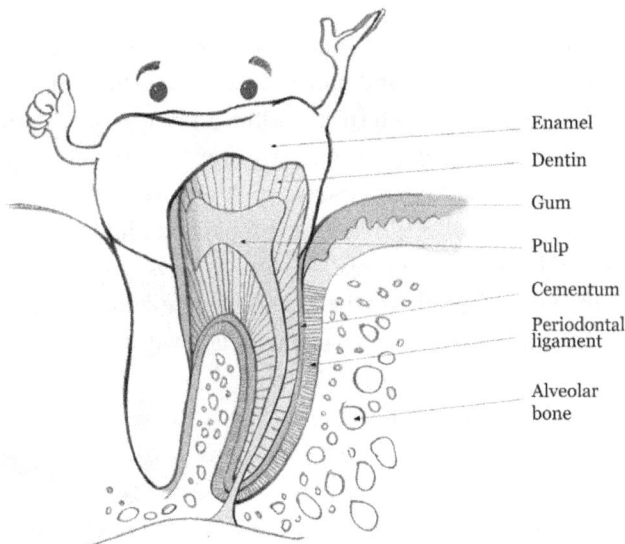

Enamel

Dentin

Gum

Pulp

Cementum

Periodontal ligament

Alveolar bone

teeth come into contact with. It is a shield protecting the tooth, withstanding wear and tear for its lifetime. The enamel is also the hardest substance found in the human body, much harder than our bones! It contains no nerves or blood supply, and is therefore an insensitive layer.

While the enamel is built tough to tolerate lifelong usage, it is, unfortunately, not a substance that the body can replenish or repair, unlike nails or hair, or even bone for that matter. Once the enamel is lost, it is gone forever! And when that happens, the fortress of the tooth is breached, making its inner layers vulnerable to attack.

Beneath the protective layer of enamel is a softer layer known as dentin or dentine (depending on which side of the Atlantic you are from). While the dentin is not as hard or insensitive as the enamel, it is the second layer of defense for the susceptible core of the tooth, and can transmit sensations to the core through fine tubular channels. If your tooth yelps at cold or sweet foods, you can blame this layer!

The innermost part—the core—is called the pulp, containing the blood and nerve supply of the tooth. The blood nourishes the tooth from within, and the moisture helps keep the structure resilient and capable of withstanding the pounding that accompanies chewing. As for the nerves in the pulp, many believe that God probably added them as an afterthought, keeping dentists' interests in mind!

Damage to the pulp is what results in agonizing toothaches: the pain can be so severe that one is left with no choice but to make a dash for the dental clinic!

The tooth has strong supporting structures that hold it entrenched in the jawbone. The gums are the superficial part of this system, while the periodontal ligament acts like a suspension to anchor the teeth in their bony sockets.

This ligament stretches between the jawbone surrounding the socket, and the roots of the teeth. The cementum is a protective layer covering the roots, and 'cements' the periodontal ligament into them.

A Set of Teeth: Many Hands Make Light Work

Teeth, just like the fingers of our hand, act as a single unit. Each tooth has a specific function, and the sum total of all their performances is what makes the entire set an efficient entity. Just as we need the full complement of fingers for the hand to carry out its tasks, we need *all* our teeth to act as a single functional component of the digestive tract.

If the teeth didn't perform their duties, we would be forced to modify our diet to eat only soft food. This would affect our daily nutritional needs, and digestion would suffer, leading to a cascading effect on our overall health. Not to forget, loss of teeth results in poor speech... and toothless smiles look good only on babies!

Any efficient machine is the sum total of its parts. The body is an incredible mechanism, honed to perfection. When we understand the pivotal role of each tooth, the need to hold on to them becomes very apparent.

Given their undeniable importance, teeth need oodles of nurture and care. Visiting the dentist regularly keeps them fighting fit!

Chapter 3

Oral Hygiene:
Brush off Your Worries

Abu l-Hasan, or Ziryab, as he was popularly known in Spain's Andalusian court of Cordoba, was popular among the medieval swish set as a musician and stylist. He is credited with being the inventor of many modern lifestyle concepts we take for granted, like dressing according to the vagaries of the season. He emphasized the need for not just clothes and hairdos, but also personal hygiene practices like bathing twice daily, especially in the hot Spanish summer!

Obviously, Ziryab would also be credited with inventing the world's first toothpaste as a part of his vision for maintaining one's personal hygiene! Though we do not know the exact concoction of this ancient toothpaste, it was rumoured to be 'useful and pleasant to taste'.

Today, it is usually kids who decide which toothpaste enters the household, depending on the power of the influence a TV advertisement has had on their young, impressionable minds. Commercials can be pretty economical with the truth, making them an iffy guide in the choice of our toothbrushes and toothpastes.

So, let's explore the reality about how far we have come from the Cordoban courts, in the evolution of oral hygiene practices!

Oral Hygiene: Clean and Clear

Broadly speaking, the term 'oral hygiene' describes all the processes you should follow in the cleansing routine of your mouth. Typically, it includes rinsing, tooth brushing and flossing.

Rinsing

Q. Which is the simplest, cheapest and most effective mouthwash?

A. Plain water!

Rinsing one's mouth after every meal—even after a wholesome food item like an apple—is a great habit in maintaining oral health. In fact, except for plain water, a good rule of thumb is that for anything you ingest, be it a beverage or a sweetmeat, you need to flush out its residues.

Rinsing, in a simple and mechanical manner, eliminates most of the food that remains in the mouth, or sticks to the teeth. As such, this action needs no special equipment, and is easily accomplished. Given the deadly effects of food particles clinging to the teeth, do make the effort to drag yourself to the washbasin each time you've finished eating or drinking something!

Then there are mouthwashes. A mouthwash, or mouth rinse, is any liquid that you can swish around inside your mouth before spitting it out. They've come a long way since the olden days when wine, or even human urine, was used to cleanse the mouth!

Presently, several mouthwashes—falling into the 'cosmetic' category—are commercially available over the counter. Containing an antiseptic ingredient, along with different flavours and colours, many are alcohol-based. They work by killing off the bacteria found in dental plaque, leaving behind a feeling of freshness in the mouth, and a temporary reprieve from bad breath.

But they have a flip side! They tend to kill off all the germs in the mouth, both the bad and the good—this can upset the delicate balance and allow the baddies to come back with a vengeance. Moreover, there are concerns about the long-term damage caused to our delicate mouth tissues by the alcohol in mouthwashes. Finally, regular use of several specific brands can stain our teeth, which could actually act as a medium for bacteria to grow on. Therefore, it is best to avoid chemical mouthwashes as a daily practice, and definitely not as a substitute for toothbrushing and flossing!

Your dentist can prescribe mouthwashes in certain situations. Those with fluoride content are popular in protecting against dental caries, especially for people with a high tendency for that affliction. This is because fluoride strengthens tooth enamel against acid attack, and fights bacteria too.

Anti-plaque rinses contain chemicals that kill mouth bacteria, or suppress their growth. These are usually recommended when oral hygiene by brushing and flossing is not feasible—typically in the case of physically, mentally or medically compromised people, for whom such activities are tasks in themselves.

Dentists also request the use of mouthwashes after certain surgical procedures when toothbrushing is suspended during the healing period. Occasionally, mouth ulcers or injuries react during toothbrushing, and the dentist may prescribe a short course of mouth rinses till they heal.

Brushing

Many ancient scriptures, much before Ziryab invented the toothpaste, carry references to oral hygiene rituals. In the East, many communities still use neem or acacia twigs (called 'datun') as part of their morning ablutions. The Prophet Muhammad encouraged the habit of chewing miswak twigs to clean the teeth, a practice that is still followed.

While datun or miswak has cleansing properties, the toothbrush is a far more popular and effective way of brushing away one's oral hygiene worries!

Like most inventions in the past, the Chinese are credited with devising the world's first toothbrush, made of ox-bone and hog hair. Soon, the toothbrush became a matter of social status, and handles of ivory were coveted. It is now unthinkable that until the twentieth century, the entire family and friends shared the same toothbrush!

Modern toothbrushes are made with nylon bristles, and plastic handles (the use of ivory is thankfully banned, internationally). Depending on the thickness of each individual bristle, they are sold in soft, medium and hard versions. While the first two are good for routine brushing, hard brushes are only suited to cleaning artificial dentures, as they are too severe on the gums and teeth.

The main role of the toothbrush is to remove the dental plaque constantly building up on our teeth, thus keeping the surfaces free of bacteria, and restraining germ-induced damage. Here are a few tips on getting it right!

Toothbrushing is recommended twice daily, once in the morning as soon as you are up (perish the thought of that bed tea!), and once just before you tumble into bed at night. Brushing in the morning helps clean the accumulation of plaque formed through the night, and it also freshens the breath. Your morning cuppa will definitely taste better after brushing! Brushing at night, too, is a must. It not only removes the remnants of dinner from the teeth, but also reduces the bacteria accumulated on them. This is vital, as our teeth are more vulnerable to germ attacks at night due to the lack of our beneficial saliva while we sleep.

To do a good job, you need to brush for two to three minutes. Anything less would be an incomplete job, while any more can injure your gums and teeth. Please brush gently! The key word is 'brush', which is a gentle movement. (Leave the scrubbing and scouring for toilet bowls and kitchen vessels!)

Whenever we tell our patients that there are numerous scientific techniques for brushing teeth, we get bewildered looks and they think we're kidding! We give you some handy tips on good brushing skills:

- Keep your elbow parallel to the ground while brushing, to minimize the force of movement.
- Please remember, you do not need to use the entire might of the arm, just a gentle roll of the wrist—we are removing just soft plaque and food residues.
- Divide the mouth into four quarters, and clean each so that no tooth is left unattended.
- The bristles of the toothbrush need to move vertically on both, the outer and inner surfaces of your teeth (that is, facing the lip/cheek and the tongue/palate). Rolling the wrists while brushing enables the correct movement.
- It is a common mistake to brush horizontally across these surfaces—small, circular movements of the brush are preferable to horizontal brushing.

- It would help further if the toothbrush can be angled at forty-five degrees to your teeth, to enable starting from the gum margins, but this may not be easy at the beginning. Keep trying!
- On the chewing surfaces, a back-and-forth movement works best.
- Don't neglect the inner surfaces of the upper and lower front teeth! Hold the brush vertically to use an outward pull stroke on these parts.
- Many of us struggle to keep the cheek-facing surfaces of our molars clean, as we feel there isn't enough space for the brush to move. We park the blame on the size and shape of the toothbrush! A simple remedy is to close the mouth a bit after inserting it—this way the cheek relaxes and creates room for easy movement of the brush.

Flossing

Let's say you just finished brushing your teeth, and did a great job. How would you react if we told you that you have cleaned only 60 per cent of your teeth, and the rest is still teeming with plaque? You would probably throw the brush at us!

So, let's break it to you gently...

Toothbrushing is really effective when it comes to cleaning three out of the five surfaces of every tooth. It works great on the lip/cheek-facing surfaces, the tongue/palate-facing surfaces, and on the chewing/biting surfaces. All of these are clearly visible, and relatively easy to deal with.

But, teeth have two other surfaces—those in contact with their immediate neighbours on either side. These are called the interdental surfaces, and because they are sheltered, they are also relatively less exposed to the natural cleansing effects of saliva—besides, they remain untouched by a toothbrush. While you cannot really see them, the mouth bacteria have no such problem! They are delighted to occupy these surfaces, and to initiate cavity formation and gum disease.

Our main weapon to deal with these hidden zones is dental floss—a simple thin nylon thread, packaged as a spool in a plastic casing, and with or without a waxy coating. You can stretch a bit of floss between the fingers of two hands, and this taut section can easily pass through the gap between two adjacent teeth. Keeping the floss tightly stretched, you can scrape the plaque off these interdental surfaces, then move on to clean the next gap, and so on, till all the teeth are done.

Flossing is recommended once daily, and is best accomplished at night before bedtime, when you are least rushed. For those who have never flossed, it can seem like a daunting task. There is a learning curve to it, but it is well worth the effort. Here are some helpful hints:

- You will need about 18-inches of floss to clean all the teeth.
- In the beginning, break the routine into smaller tasks.
- Start with learning about your front teeth, using a mirror to help guide the floss between them.
- In a few days, you will be familiar with the operation. You can then floss the next few teeth, say, till the premolars. Stay at this level till you get it right.
- Lastly, you can graduate to the molars—which poses the highest level of difficulty. By now, you will know how to manage the hand positions to reach right to the back of the mouth.
- Use a sawing motion to guide the floss into the tight

spaces between the teeth. Don't try to snap the floss into the interdental spaces—this increases the chances of the floss injuring the gums, and causing them to bleed.

- Remember that there are two surfaces to be flossed in each gap between two adjacent teeth. Once you insert the floss into the gap, wrap it around one of the teeth to scrape it clean. Then wrap it around the adjacent tooth to repeat the same exercise. Exit this 'interdental' space only when both surfaces are done.
- Use a fresh section of floss for each interdental space, so that the germs from a soiled section do not get transported into a new space.
- You can floss under bridgework too—with a floss threader, which is like a plastic needle, to get the floss into that space.
- If you have large hands, it may be difficult to floss the back teeth. Try using a floss holder, which can simplify the situation.

The Oral Hygiene Kit: Tools for Trade

Maintained Manual Toothbrush

It goes without saying that your toothbrush is a personal hygiene tool, and should never be shared! After use, it ought to be cleaned thoroughly, and allowed to dry. Once dry, it must be kept enclosed within a plastic cap, and never left unprotected, as bacteria from the bathroom/toilet may grow on it.

It is best to change your toothbrush every two to three months, as the bristles start losing shape. If it wears out or

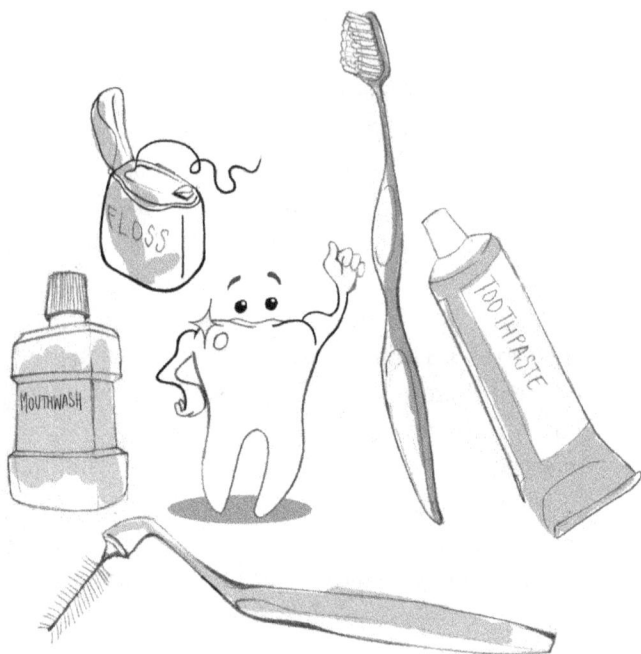

'flowers' much before the estimated time, it means that you are applying more force than necessary while brushing.

On the other hand, if there is hardly any wear after three months, then the brushing may not be effective enough, or the brush not used twice a day.

Electrical and Battery-operated Toothbrush

Modern day trends have ensured that even the humble manual toothbrush morphs into a motorized one! Way back in 1954, Dr Philippe-Guy Woog from Switzerland invented the Broxodont, an electric toothbrush, as he wanted to revolutionize our oral hygiene practices. With their oscillatory or rotational movement they soon gained popularity in the West.

Today, these brushes are battery-operated to avoid the possibility of electric shock. Most of them employ a circular or rotational movement, and are extremely effective in cleaning plaque away from the teeth and gums. Some are also equipped with a two-minute timer to help you keep track of your brushing time.

They have an added advantage: one cannot apply excessive pressure while brushing, else the brush stops running! This is a great feature, as most of us tend to scrub our teeth or apply undue force on the manual toothbrush, assuming that we are cleaning better.

As with the manual toothbrush, the brush head of the battery-operated one needs to be cleaned thoroughly, kept protected, and needs replacement every three months. They are a great boon for folks with suboptimal manual dexterity, or for physically or mentally challenged people who find it difficult to use a manual toothbrush efficiently. They also work well for those undergoing orthodontic treatment.

A recent development is the 'ultrasonic' toothbrush: it uses ultrasound waves that vibrate at a very high frequency, to remove dental plaque from the teeth. Most also combine a motor for the rotary movement, to work in a synergistic manner.

Dentifrice

A dentifrice is any substance used in combination with a toothbrush to clean the teeth—it could be a powder, paste, gel or liquid. Toothpowders and toothpastes are the examples most familiar to us.

In India, a number of communities use the ground husks of grains with or without salt, as a cleaning medium. This coarse mixture is rubbed on the teeth with the finger. Even today, there are people who use tobacco as a tooth cleanser. Most such powders are extremely abrasive, and cause a great deal of tooth wear. Therefore, dentists don't recommend any of these powder dentifrices.

If one is marooned on an island, and could choose between a floating toothbrush and a tube of toothpaste, one ought to choose the toothbrush! Yet, most of us won't be satisfied if we don't use toothpaste on it.

While toothpastes are highly advertised, with many claims and counterclaims, most of them are equally good. They work on a pretty standard formula, with a few additions and deletions! All of them combine fine abrasives, detergents, flavouring, and colouring agents. Some add antibacterial ingredients, or additions like salt, neem, etc. Others are specifically designed to counter tooth sensitivity, containing one of several desensitizing agents.

One of the main ingredients to have helped toothpaste become an integral element of oral hygiene is fluoride—these salts have been proven to fight tooth decay. They strengthen the enamel, making it more resistant to bacterial acid attack, and they come with their own antibacterial properties as well. Except for geographical areas where the natural concentration of fluoride is high in drinking water, fluoridated toothpaste is highly recommended for all ages above six.

Some toothpastes, containing ingredients with a sustained antibacterial effect under 'ideal' or 'test' conditions, claim to offer twelve or even twenty-four hour protection against cavities. As it is impractical to replicate those conditions in our mouths, it would be prudent to ignore these claims! But, what *can* give you good and simple round-the-clock protection is if you brush well, eat sensibly, and watch less TV!

There is even a correct technique for applying the

toothpaste on the toothbrush. Contrary to the visuals seen in advertisements, it is not to be left merely on the top of the brush, but to be pushed well into the bristles to affect a sustained release throughout the three-minute cycle. Else, the entire blob would get stuck on the first tooth as you start brushing!

Tongue Cleaner

The tongue is crawling with the same bacteria found on the teeth. Your oral health routine is incomplete without a good tongue-clean. Sadly, this aspect of mouth hygiene is often neglected. Even if you've brushed your teeth very thoroughly, when you miss cleaning your tongue, the germs inhabiting it can hop onto the gums and teeth very easily, re-populating them both!

The simplest way to clean the tongue is by brushing it down with your regular toothbrush, or with another kept exclusively for the purpose. No toothpaste is needed, but do remember to stiffen your tongue while cleaning it to prevent a gagging sensation.

Better still, one can use plastic tongue cleaners/scrapers. It is best to avoid the metallic versions, even stainless steel versions, as they are prone to corrosion, which might not necessarily be noticed by the naked eye. Additionally, the metal abrades the delicate taste buds, and can damage them in the long run.

Toothpick

Our ancestors most probably used the toothpick when they were hunters and gatherers to remove fibrous meat stuck between their teeth.

The indulgences of ancient royalty also meant that they

would use golden toothpicks, as did the Mesopotamian kings.

While the humble toothpick is much maligned in polite social circles, it can help dislodge large food particles stuck between teeth. One needs to use it very carefully and gently to avoid injuring the gums. Etiquette demands covering one's mouth when using it in the presence of others. If you find yourself regularly picking your teeth, you need to get your dentist to fix the cause of the issue.

Interdental Brush

An interdental brush works much better, and is a safer option than toothpicks for removing food particles from interdental spaces. Some of us may have large gaps between our teeth, or gums that have receded substantially. Floss may not clean such areas effectively, and it is here, too, that interdental brushes are most useful. Imagine a toothpick coated with soft bristles—that's what an interdental brush looks like! It keeps the gaps between teeth free of plaque and reduces tartar formation in those areas too.

Oral Irrigator

This is a home-care device that uses a pulsating stream of pressurized water to remove deep-seated plaque from inaccessible areas, such as the interdental gaps, and from below the gum line. These are most useful for people undergoing orthodontic treatment, who find it difficult to brush effectively. Not as effective as toothbrushing and flossing, but oral irrigators can be easier to use than floss. They are also useful for cleaning under complete dentures which are fixed in place over dental implants.

Chewing Gum

Labdanum, a plant-based resin, finds a mention in the Bible as a remedy for bad breath—it was probably the world's first chewing gum! The ancient Greeks chewed another resin, mastic, as a breath freshener.

Chewing gum is an effective way of freshening one's breath and keeping teeth and gums healthy. It helps in cleaning our teeth surfaces, and stimulates salivary secretion, which adds to protection against cavities.

It is best, however, to avoid sweetened gum, as it releases sugary content, exposing the teeth to bacterial attack. Xylitol, an artificial sweetener, is a preferred ingredient of many chewing gums, and has an antibacterial effect too.

We also need to regulate the duration for which the gum is chewed, as prolonged chewing tends to increase wear and tear of the teeth, and can damage the joint of our jaws as well over time.

So, there is a vast armamentarium at our disposal for keeping our teeth healthy, and to prevent cavities and gum disease. Choose your weapons well, and brush away your worries!

Chapter 4

Sugar:
Food for Rot

Let's start with a very bold statement: if we had continued to eat what we did in the caves, we would not have cavities!

Find it hard to digest? Consider this: dental caries is, largely, a human syndrome, and can easily fall into the category of a 'lifestyle' disease. Tooth decay is virtually unheard of in animals, who stick to eating what nature intended them to!

Junk Food: The Ills of Evolution

Food is the essential fuel that keeps our bodies going. Eating right is fundamental to maintenance of overall health. Our diet provides all the nutrients needed to keep our system ticking, and obviously—depending on what we eat—will have both positive and negative effects on our wellbeing.

The change in our food habits, over the years, has also been highly influenced by the media, which exhorts us to consume various specific food items, which either promise great health benefits, or are imbued with a 'cool' quotient! Many of these advertisements—even though the claims are usually unsubstantiated—target children and young adults, who are the most impressionable.

As a result, our diet has shifted from the healthy

nutritious food we ate, to the more processed and unhealthy foods available in the market. Just a few decades ago, before television brought all the processed junk goodies into our dining room, we were content with homemade food and snacks.

The same influences have ensured that dental decay today is the one of the most rampant diseases affecting humankind, as what we eat and drink impacts our teeth directly.

Spawning Bacteria and Plaque: Germ Warfare

In the earlier sections, we learnt that the tooth enamel is the hardest in the body, with strong mineral armour, much like a fortress. Our saliva works as a moat, keeping intruders away, and has its own version of 'moat-monsters' to attack them.

We will soon learn a few things about the enemy, and its wily ways (see Chapter Seven). We will learn how bacteria form a coalition to generate plaque, which gains a foothold on our teeth to catalyze the process of destruction. We will also follow the natural history of cavity formation when germs are given undisturbed quality time to launch their attack.

The irony is that *we* are helping the enemy! Who feeds the bad bacteria that harm our teeth? Us! Haven't we been told, right from our childhood, not to eat too much chocolate, else we would get toothache? Yet, not many of us have realized that it's not just chocolates that are the villains causing cavities and bad oral health. If we understand that the term 'chocolate' was denoted in the broadest sense, encompassing all sweets, we can conclude that the main culprit is sugar!

How Sugar Facilitates Tooth Decay: In a Ferment

Sugar is technically an easily fermentable carbohydrate. What does this mean?

Most of us are aware of the phenomenon of fermentation, a simple example being the setting of milk into yoghurt or curd. Here, bacteria are introduced in milk, and they break down its sugar content (lactose) to release lactic acid, which emits the sourness in curd.

Therefore, the process of fermentation requires bacterial action on a sugar-containing substance (the by-product of which is an acid) or an alcohol (as in wine fermentation), or a gas (such as carbon dioxide during the fermentation process of beer-brewing).

As far as tooth decay is concerned, the most worrying by-product of bacterial fermentation in the mouth is acid!

Our diet has three major nutritional components: carbohydrates, proteins and fats. We know our carbs, don't we? Fitness enthusiasts will vouch for the ability of carbs to confer instant energy, but they also feed a huge dose of calories to your waistline! And if that were not enough, they feed the cavity-causing germs lurking in our mouths!

We consume a large amount of food that falls in the category of fermentable carbohydrates. All of them are sugary and starchy and can be easily broken down—both by bacteria in our mouths, and by chemicals in our saliva called enzymes. This process is technically known as 'glycolysis'.

The one ingredient in our food, which these decay-causing bacteria adore, is sugar! Just as most of us enjoy our sugar-highs, so do these critters!

The dental plaque covering our teeth is full of bacteria waiting for such food. The moment we eat sugary and starchy stuff, enzymes in our saliva start breaking them down into simpler sugars.

So, whether it's a sinfully sweet Black Forest cake or a healthier apple, the leftovers on our teeth will all be meals for the germs. The mouth-bacteria gobble them up with greed, initiating the process of fermentation. If these acids are allowed to remain on the teeth, they start dissolving the hard tooth enamel and accelerate the process of tooth decay.

Causes of Tooth Decay

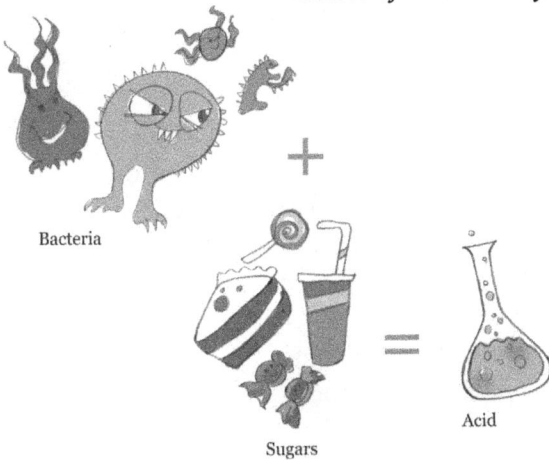

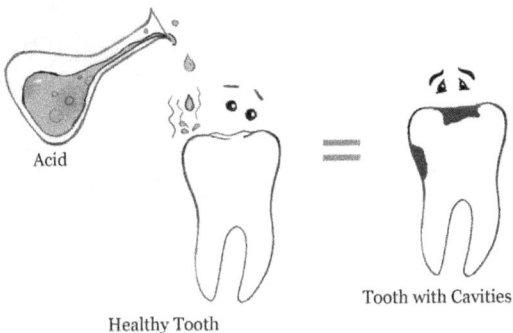

Bacteria

Sugars

Acid

Acid

Healthy Tooth

Tooth with Cavities

The Sugar Diet: Unmasking the Villains

All carbs that can be broken down easily by the germs in our mouth, into sugar or sucrose, and eventually the simplest sugar—glucose—are bad for our teeth! If ever there were a dental award for 'best actor in a negative role', the honours would go to the arch criminal—$C_{12}H_{22}O_{11}$—more commonly known as sucrose (a kind of sugar)!

In our modern diets, sugar is easily available for oral acid fermentation from the following foods:

- Chocolates and sweetmeats
- Cakes, pastries and biscuits
- Fresh/preserved fruit and fruit juices
- Honey, jams, molasses and sweet sauces
- Ice creams and sweetened aerated drinks
- Sweetened milk beverages
- Boiled sweets, candies and jujubes
- Sweetened tea/coffee
- Peppermints/after-mints
- Processed ready-made cereals

In addition, starchy foods like rice and other cereals, too, eventually break down into sugar. Try keeping a piece of bread in your mouth awhile, and the taste changes to sweet as the oral enzymes begin breaking the starch into sugar. Fortunately, this is a more lengthy process, hence these complex carbs are relatively safer.

Joining hands with sugar are acidic foods, which also promote the dissolving of tooth enamel. Some prime examples are:

- Citrus juices
- Cola drinks

- Pickles
- Vinegar

All of these create a highly acidic environment in the mouth, which potentiates the damage caused by sugar.

Luckily, there are many food items that are either 'cavity-neutral' or have 'anti-cavity' properties. These protective foods work in different ways:

- Some raw vegetables like cucumber or celery, and other high-fiber produce like beansprouts, promote the flow of saliva, bringing its protective qualities into action with a detergent-like effect in your mouth.
- A few foods, due to their alkaline nature, have the capacity to neutralize acids. Examples are cheddar cheese, green leafy vegetables, almonds, walnuts and carrots. Still or uncarbonated water is also effective.
- Dairy products—unsweetened milk, yoghurt or curd, and cheese—contain calcium and phosphorus, which help remineralize early impairment caused by acid attack. Try to include them in your diet.
- Antibacterial foods include black and green tea, with compounds called polyphenols. Shiitake mushrooms and wasabi, both favourites in Oriental cuisine, also fight cavity-causing germs. And a surprise inclusion: cocoa! The tannins in cocoa are anti-cavity, so you could opt for some bitter chocolate without too much guilt!

Balancing the Sugar Diet: Have Your Cake and Eat It Too!

The good news is that to keep your teeth healthy, you do *not* have to withdraw from all the goodies and lead a monastic life! While sugar has become an integral part of our lives, we can learn to manage its consumption to minimize its ill effects on our teeth. There are many variable factors, which determine the hazard-level of our sugar intake, and if we can load these in our favour, we can have the best of both worlds.

Consuming Optimal Quantities

Obviously, it helps to cut down on the total quantity of sugar consumed on any given day. Not only will you benefit in terms of a reduction in cavity formation, but also, avoiding the heavy overdose of empty calories improves your overall health.

Checking the Frequency of Consumption

A major factor contributing to tooth decay: every time our teeth are subjected to sugar, an acid attack is inflicted on them in about half-an-hour. If we limit the number of times we consume anything sugary, we curtail the number of acid attacks.

For example, from the cavity point-of-view, it would be better to gorge on a large bar of chocolate at one go, rather than to break it up into multiple chunks to be eaten several times during the day! For the same reason, it is better to plan three or four meals in a day, and to strictly avoid snacking in between. And if you do want something for the elevenses, snack on the anti-cavity food mentioned above!

Making Note of the Nature and Texture of Food

Sweet foods come in various forms, and some are more harmful than others. The crucial point is the amount of time it spends in contact with the teeth. For example, while munching nutritious raisins is healthier than eating highly sweetened and sticky chocolates, they too release their inherent sweetness over an extended period, by sticking to our teeth.

The exposure from this slow-releasing sugar, therefore, becomes as undesirable, for kids, as chomping on an éclair. They, who prefer lollipops, hard candied sweets or jujubes, are at a higher risk of getting cavities, as these release their juices over prolonged spans. Grateful germs eat the sticky residues at their leisure, increasing injury to the teeth.

In contrast, a sweet drink doesn't remain for long in the mouth, and the salivary action helps in quickly flushing it away before it can cause serious harm.

The bottom line: while you may love the sweet taste lingering in your mouth after eating that deliciously gooey mousse, you may be better off drinking that chocolate milkshake instead. Even better, some still water perhaps?

Balancing the Aggravating or Mitigating Factors

The consumption of sweet foods can be accompanied by others, which can either neutralize the effects of sugar, or enhance them.

The detrimental effects of sugary foods can be made worse by combining them with acidic food or drinks, as they double the likely ruin of our teeth.

Smokers generally try to mask mouth odours by sucking on breath mints or mentholated boiled sweets after every smoke. The teeth suffer a double whammy here: as it is, smoking depresses the immunity of the mouth, and then a heavy sugar load follows. The result: rampant cavity formation!

As a nation, we harbour a sweet-rich culture. So, while it's not possible to forbid our children from consuming sweets, we can ask that they combine them with their main meals, when the salivary flow is at its best and helps in diluting the effect of the sugary food. They must, of course, follow that up with brushing their teeth.

Culturally, we tend to eat with the hand, which necessitates a visit to the washbasin after a meal. This is a great opportunity to rinse the mouth thoroughly: it removes most of the food crumbs clinging to the teeth, and dilutes any sweet residue around. While rinsing the mouth is not as efficient as tooth brushing, it may be more easily doable, and is a valuable addition to our arsenal.

Sugar substitutes are effective in lowering our overall sugar consumption—sweeteners like sorbitol or xylitol are freely available, and can sweeten your daily cuppa. Xylitol, a naturally occurring chemical, found in many fruits and berries, and also in corn, is now a common ingredient in sugar-free gums, lozenges, etc. It carries the additional benefit of stimulating salivary secretion, and helps in repairing areas of acid attack.

While we cannot dream of going back to the caves and escaping cavities, we can, with a little effort, manage our diet wisely enough to overcome the adverse effects of sweet nothings. We Indians *are* genetically prone to diabetes mellitus, and apart from escaping the pain caused by cavities, a sensible approach to sugar consumption can also stave off the tendency for acquiring the disease. Now, isn't that a sweet incentive?

Chapter 5

Nutrition:
Eat to Live

An effective way to manage dental health is by eating a healthy balanced diet. Good nutrition is essential not only for the maintenance of our teeth but also for the optimal functioning of the entire body.

A Balanced Diet for Teeth: Chew on This

More often than not we forget that the primary role of teeth is for chewing or mastication. They break down our food mechanically, so as to make the rest of the chemical process of digestion easier.

We often cite a simple example in our dental practice, using a coconut as an analogy. Just as one prepares a coconut for grinding in a processor by first breaking it and then scraping it, similarly, our teeth accomplish the initial stage of processing the digestion of our food. Had we put the entire coconut into the processor, it would heat up and eventually lose the

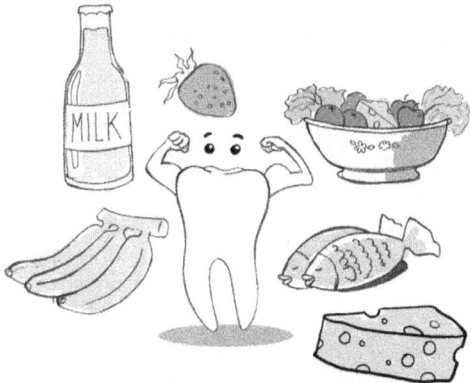

battle. Similarly, the food that we ingest has to be chewed thoroughly, and made into a paste with the assistance of the saliva in our mouth. If we gulp down our food without chewing it, our digestive system could fold up!

Many of us with missing teeth think we are managing fine, but remain unaware of the long-term damage being caused by their absence. If the teeth aren't around to do their job well, the digestive system will protest. If the digestive system fails to cooperate with us, it is unlikely we will ever be healthy!

Dentists frequently see patients who are overweight. One of the reasons is that they have lost some of their chewing teeth, and not had them replaced. Tooth-loss induces a change towards an unhealthy diet, because one tends to avoid nutritious foods which need to be chewed well, such as raw vegetables or nuts. You opt for softer diets instead—usually rich in carbs or fat—as they can be swallowed without much mastication.

Apart from a balanced intake of the primaries—carbohydrates, proteins and fats—we need a host of other nutrients to keep the system ticking. Let's take a look at some that are pertinent to our teeth and bones.

Calcium

This mineral is the building block of our teeth and bones, and we need to ensure that our diet is not calcium-deficient in any way. Dairy products are rich sources, so please don't skimp on your milk, cheese, yoghurt and curd! You can also get calcium from green leafy veggies like spinach, and from soya, fish and whole grains like ragi/nachni (finger millet).

Expectant women need healthy doses of calcium to meet its increased demand during pregnancy. It is important to ensure sufficiency of calcium intake in the case of children, too, for the proper development of their teeth and bones

Milk teeth start forming in the foetus, and continue to develop outside the womb. The permanent teeth begin their genesis soon after birth, and complete their evolution sequentially by the age of twelve. Once the formation of teeth is complete, their calcium requirement is over—therefore, adults needn't worry about its deficiency affecting their teeth (but they still need to get enough of it for their bones!).

Phosphorus

Along with calcium, phosphorus is essential for the formation of teeth and bones. Dietary sources include eggs, dairy products, oily fish, meat, beans and soya.

Vitamin D

This vitamin is necessary for regulating the uptake of calcium and phosphorus by our teeth and bones, and is therefore a crucial ingredient in their formation. Foods rich in this resource include milk, cottage cheese, fish such as salmon, and eggs. A good twenty-minute exposure to sunlight also helps the body generate this vitamin naturally.

Fluoride

This salt strengthens the tooth enamel, making it more resistant to acid attacks by bacteria. It occurs naturally in well water, and since seawater contains considerable quantities of fluoride, most seafood is rich in it too. Tea is also a good source.

Vitamin C

This is essential to maintain the tissues anchoring our teeth within the jawbone, and to keep the blood vessels healthy. It is also an antioxidant, which protects our tissues from harmful chemicals. A deficiency of this vitamin can lead to bleeding gums and weak teeth. Luckily, vitamin C is abundantly present in many food sources, such as bell peppers, citrus fruits, gooseberries, guavas, etc.

Others

Several other nutrients impact the health of our teeth, bones, and other soft tissues of the mouth, like the mouth lining.

Zinc, vitamin A, all the B vitamins and omega-3 fats are essential for keeping the mouth tissues and our immune system healthy. Some trace elements like molybdenum have sundry anti-cavity properties. Vegetarians, and the increasing followers of veganism, are likely to manifest deficiencies in certain vitamins like riboflavin, and specifically vitamin B12 that is found only in an animal-based diet. It's best to supplement their requirement with multivitamins to compensate.

If the vegetarian's diet is tilted more towards fruits, then the potential to form dental caries is even higher, as their fructose content is an easy feed for decay-causing bacteria. Those on a total vegetable/fruit diet, or on other weight-loss food plans, are also vulnerable to oral health issues.

It must be remembered that any change in an optimally balanced diet can affect our overall health and also our oral wellbeing. A diet that includes green leafy vegetables, nuts, lentils, seeds, eggs, dairy products, fish and lean meat bestow the whole range of nutrients needed by us. Eating raw, crunchy vegetables lends good exercise for the teeth, and also cleans them in the bargain! Needless to say, limiting our intake of sugary and processed foods can spare us painful cavities.

Eating right is crucial to dental health—our teeth are designed to last a lifetime, let's not eat them out of business!

Chapter 6

Milk Teeth:
No Kidding

Polyphyodonts are lucky! This term refers to creatures that grow many sets of teeth over their lifetime—such as crocodiles, sharks and even some mammals like elephants. We humans, unfortunately, are diphyodonts. In other words, we grow only two sets of teeth—milk teeth as children and permanent teeth that need to last for the rest of our lives.

The Rise of Milk Teeth: A Tooth Is Born

Our baby teeth are called milk teeth, due to their colour, which is milk white. They start forming even before we are born—in the sixth week of the embryo the tooth 'bud' germinates, and continues to grow like a flower till it erupts out of the gums. They are also called deciduous teeth, as they fall off at their appointed time.

There is a predictable sequence to the teething process, or 'eruption', as it is technically called. The first teeth to erupt are usually the lower front teeth, or incisors, at around six months of age. After this, the others follow in stages, and the eruption of all twenty milk teeth is normally complete by the age of two years. The last to erupt is usually the upper second grinder or molar teeth. (Refer to the image: 'Milk Teeth Timetable'.)

Each jaw holds ten milk teeth—four incisors, two canines and four molars.

Generally, teeth appear in pairs, first in the lower jaw and then in the upper. Just as they follow a sequence of eruption, there is a pattern for their shedding or exfoliation.

Interestingly, it has been observed that girls receive and lose their teeth earlier than boys!

A very large percentage of children have gaps between their milk teeth, which is natural (in fact, some of these are called 'primate' spaces, reflecting their evolutionary origin). Although they cause much worry to parents, who feel the need to have them seen to, these gaps are important for the jaw to accommodate the larger permanent teeth when they arrive. Best left alone—it is wiser to worry about providing good oral care for your child instead!

The Role of Milk Teeth: They Also Serve...

'Why do my child's milk teeth need special care? Aren't they going to fall off anyway? And get replaced by spanking new permanent teeth, which are far more long lasting?'

These are familiar questions going through every parent's mind. The answers can be found in understanding the vital role of milk teeth within the overall growth and development of children.

Chewing

Children need their milk teeth to chew their food! They also need them to eat a healthy diet that needs to be well masticated; this diet includes crisp vegetables, fruit, nuts or lean meats. Often children with decayed or missing milk teeth compromise on nutritious fare, which they are unable to chew. They then start preferring high-calorie and junk foods that don't need much effort to be swallowed. Obviously, the child's overall growth will be greatly affected on account of the resulting poor nourishment.

Speech

Teeth, especially the front ones, cast a major influence on speech. Certain sounds and words are articulated clearly only due to their presence. While a childlike lisp may sound cute in the early days, children can develop serious impairment of speech if they lose their milk teeth due to neglect. This could have an adverse effect on the child's confidence and overall personality development.

Appearance

Milk teeth lend a normal and pleasant shape to the face of the child, whose appearance and confidence levels improve. This is all-important in today's world, which puts such a premium on our physical image. Children with missing teeth—especially the front ones—often seem to lack confidence in social interactions.

Space Maintenance

Milk teeth 'reserve' space in the jaw for their respective successors, the permanent teeth. If milk teeth are lost, or removed prematurely, they cannot act as guides for their followers to erupt in their rightful places. This often results in the permanent teeth emerging haphazardly, in misaligned and crooked positions.

The Rise of Permanent Teeth: Mix and Match

From the age of six years, parents need to be prepared for the permanent teeth to surface.

Some permanent teeth could crop up side-by-side with milk teeth. Most parents panic when they see the lower front permanent teeth erupting behind their corresponding milk teeth. There is usually no cause for worry, as the latter eventually drop off and the permanent ones quickly move into position.

Parents need to watch out for an important tooth—the first permanent molar—which arrives at the age of six, along with the lower permanent front teeth. It comes up right behind the last milk molar, without the loss of any milk tooth. As parents and children don't see any tooth fall, they fail to realize that this one is permanent. It usually has deep grooves on its chewing surface, which can retain food particles. Children frequently forget to brush this tooth, as it is the last in the jaw at the time. Therefore, it is customarily the first permanent tooth to decay, so parents need to be extra careful with this one.

There is a time when permanent teeth, especially the incisors, look too large on a baby's face, occupying most of the tiny countenance, and imparting a 'bunny rabbit' look! Here, we need to understand that the size of these permanent teeth will remain the same forever (except for some wear and tear with age), while the jaw and the face increase in size dramatically during spurts of growth.

Soon after, comes the 'ugly duckling stage', where kids manifest large gaps between their front teeth. Their side incisors look wonky, the front ones seem to jut out, and the upper permanent canines aren't in yet. Not beautiful at all!

But when the size of the jaw increases, and the upper canines power their way in, the teeth start looking more proportionate, and your child transforms herself from an 'ugly duckling' to a beautiful swan!

Rarely, even this growth stage may be inadequate to align the teeth well enough, in which case the child may need the help of an orthodontist to straighten them out.

It is worth noting that the onset of menarche in girls is accompanied by a growth spurt, and thereby their jaw size increases earlier than in boys, who attain maturity at a later age.

Home Care in the Pre-tooth Days: Armed to the Teeth

The important role of milk teeth in the child's overall growth means that caring for them needs to begin early!

Parents are the first caregivers of their child's oral health, and they need to keep at it till their kid is able to do a good job on her own. It is imperative to understand that oral hygiene procedures need to start even before the first milk teeth arrive. The primary check should be done as soon as the baby is born! Occasionally, newborns have rudimentary tooth-like structures at birth, which—though not harmful for the infant—often hurt the mother when nursing. Thankfully these natal teeth lack support, and usually exfoliate on their own, without much ado.

In the beginning, the baby's gum pads can be cleaned with a fresh, clean strip of soft cloth. This not only keeps the wee one's mouth hygienic, it also conditions the child to accept mouth-cleaning procedures later, which can be a boon!

Dentists play a pivotal part, and parents naturally turn to them regarding the right time to get their child across for the first dental checkup. Visit one soon after your child is born!

Baby Bottle Decay

Paediatricians and dentists advise against milk bottles, but many parents still prefer feeding their baby with it. Many a time, it is left in the mouth after the last feed, as the little one nods off to sleep. The milk is often sweetened, and the residue in the infant's mouth pools around the upper front, and the back teeth. This creates ideal conditions for the growth of bacteria, which can cause rapid tooth decay. Such tots usually end up with multiple cavities in their upper teeth and the molars, in what is known as 'milk bottle syndrome'!

Luckily, the tongue protects the lower front teeth, so these are usually spared. Of course, it is best to not use a milk bottle at all, but if parents still find this is unavoidable, they should try to minimize the harm to the teeth. After the last milk feed, clean water must replace it, so that it rinses away all damaging milk residues.

There is considerable debate on whether breast-fed babies, too, could similarly suffer tooth decay. Fortunately, breast milk carries antibodies against decay-causing germs, and it tends to flow towards the throat, without pooling in the mouth. And it's not sweetened!

Teething Troubles

Many infants experience mild soreness or pain during the teething process, when their teeth break out through the gums. Teething rings are commercially available, and can help soothe the affected areas. Alternatively, parents could dip a piece of clean cloth/gauze in ice-cold water, squeeze it dry and then press it on the gums. If the pain persists, analgesics can be given, with the paediatrician's consent.

Teething has also traditionally been associated with other disturbances, such as fever, irritability and tummy upsets: these are incidental, and not due to tooth eruption.

Home Care for Milk Teeth: Read Our Lips

Keeping your young one's teeth clean is no child's play! Here are some guidelines on how to get it spot on.

When the milk teeth start erupting, they can be cleaned with a piece of gauze. As more teeth erupt, you can use a baby toothbrush without toothpaste, or a small ring brush slipped around your fingers, to clean baby's teeth. The tongue too should be cleaned with a soft cloth or with the ring brush as far as possible.

From the age of two, as the toddler becomes capable of rinsing on his/her own, a pea-sized dollop of toothpaste (meant exclusively for children), can be used to brush their teeth.

By the same age, most kids have also formed their individual personalities and strong egos, and resist such parental efforts. While your child can be allowed to brush on his/her own to start with, you need to declare a timeout, and administer a thorough brushing yourself.

Brushing the teeth will take at least two to three minutes, so as to cover all the surfaces. The little one can sit on the parent's lap, facing forwards during this exercise; a ritual that can continue till the child is comfortable standing in front of the parent.

And please don't forget to floss! Ideally, you need to start flossing your child's teeth as soon as two adjacent ones start touching each other. With most kids, this happens around the age of two, when the milk molars are in place.

Cleaning the tongue with the toothbrush or a tongue

scraper must be done after brushing their teeth. Youngsters should be encouraged to rinse their mouth well after brushing, so that all remnants of toothpaste are eliminated.

Parents need to continue brushing their children's teeth till around the age of four, when kids normally develop the ability to take over fully.

However, till the age of six, parents still need to supervise the toothbrushing. In the morning 'rush hour', youngsters tend to skip brushing for the appointed two to three minutes. Often, the brush isn't doing much in the mouth, as the kiddie is still groggy and merely rinses the toothpaste out. Parents can ensure that no shortcuts are taken!

From age six, children can brush on their own, without parental supervision. However, the ability to floss, independently, comes only by age ten.

Dentists may also advise home use of special fluoride gels (containing stannous fluoride), or mouth rinses with sodium fluoride, if they feel that the child is at increased risk of cavity formation.

A Diet for Milk Teeth: Lick One's Chops

Good food habits need to start early! Back in Chapter Four, we explored the cardinal role of wrong dietary habits in influencing dental disease. Here is a small recap, with your child in focus.

The bombardment from various media channels, of advertisements for junk food and fizzy drinks, are invariably targeted at children, creating a need for these unhealthy foods in their impressionable minds. Therefore, instead of good old plain water, these innocents start preferring carbonated drinks, cleverly endorsed by their favourite idols. The powerful influence of television cannot be negated entirely from our lives. But conscientious parents must take the initiative to explain and inculcate healthy eating habits in their children. Once in a while, an aerated drink is fine, and will give your child a feel-good moment, but it surely should not replace water during regular meals.

Most parents are unaware of the insidious presence of sugar in their child's daily diet. While it is easily understood that chocolates are sweet, biscuits—especially cream ones that are nutritionally deficient—are often overlooked. Besides, many 'health drinks' for children include sugar, chocolate and other additives that are wrongly projected as mandatory for the child's wholesome growth and development. Milk is healthy, but not when you add sugar! While fruit juices are nutritious enough, and far better than aerated, fizzy drinks, most of them also have added sugar, making them more likely to cause tooth decay.

Of course, children also love their milkshakes, desserts and boiled sweets! Don't deprive your child by banning sweets altogether—kids will be kids! Let them eat sweets—but in moderation—preferably after a major meal, but which ought to be followed-up by brushing their teeth.

Snacking on sweet foods between meals should be discouraged, as this tends to increase the number of sugar 'hits' on the teeth. If your child does snack, try to get him to rinse his mouth well, as it may not be practical to expect him to brush after each snack.

Ideally, though, snacking between meals should be restricted to healthy food; this will not only nourish the child, but also help maintain oral hygiene. Nuts, sprouts and homemade treats are far better in their nutritional quotient than processed, ready-to-eat food items.

If the refreshment is acidic, it is important to neutralize it with alkaline food, or which is likely to bind the acids. This is why devouring a cheese or a vegetable/chicken sandwich is much better than consuming a jam sandwich! Fruits like apples, grapes and oranges are acidic, so they could be combined with major meals.

When children start attending school, a few simple precautions can ensure that they eat right. Parents should send healthy, nutritious eatables in their lunch boxes, and avoid packing junk food like biscuits and processed snacks. Keep the lunch box tooth-friendly by keeping it sugar-free.

Most children don't rinse their mouths after eating at school: instruct them to at least sip water from their bottles immediately after.

Many schools now discourage children from eating the chocolates and sweets distributed by their classmates during birthdays. They, however, will eat these goodies on the way home! You can get them to brush their teeth after reaching; else the sticky sweet particles will most likely remain on them till the next meal!

Preventive Care for Milk Teeth: Enter the Dentist!

Prevention is better than cure—so the proverb goes, and this really holds true with children and their oral health. Apart from routine dental home care, children need to be taken for regular six-monthly checkups at the dentist's.

If you take your child regularly for dental reviews, the dentist can establish a better rapport with him under pleasant conditions! We advise parents to also take their children along on some of their own dental visits. That way they get acquainted, not just with the dentist and the staff, but also with the smells, sounds and feel of the clinic. A sense of familiarity builds up, which often quells any apprehension children may have when they are due to visit the dentist.

If we drag a child to the dental clinic only when he has a painful tooth, a negative association is drawn with the visit as he may need extensive treatment. This makes the child shy away from going to the dentist in future, and which eventually leads to neglect of his dental problems.

During the inspection, all the teeth, gums and the entire mouth can be examined closely. Cavities would be detected early enough to necessitate only minimal treatment. The condition of the gums is observed, and the alignment of teeth assessed. Encroaching problems can be identified and nipped in the bud. The status of the milk teeth and their erupting permanent successors are closely monitored. Occasionally, the dentist may recommend X-rays to detect hidden cavities, or to check the budding permanent teeth within the jaws. Of course, the dentist will also reinforce the need for the right food habits and the correct regimen for oral hygiene.

Many procedures are available for preventing the onset of dental problems, and your dentist can advise such as are specifically suitable for your child. These can ward off tooth decay, gum disease and even some teeth alignment issues.

Fluoride

One of the primary concerns about children's teeth is the occurrence of caries. Fluoride, with its anti-bacterial component, is a potent weapon in our battle against this. It works against cavity-causing germs, and alters the mineral structure of tooth enamel, making it more resistant to acid attack. Fluoride can also help in repairing areas of acid attack through a process known as remineralization.

Fluoride salts, at varying concentrations, are naturally present in drinking water, but the optimal strength needed for it to exert any anti-cavity effect is one part-per-million (ppm). In India, only 200 districts in nearly fifteen states have drinking water matching up to this requirement. Conversely, residents in areas with water containing excessive fluoride levels may develop adverse effects such as fluorosis, which damages the teeth and bones.

Please check with your local authorities about the fluoride concentration of your drinking water. If you live in a region with a deficient level of fluoride, your child can use fluoridated toothpaste after the age of six, which delivers its anti-cavity benefits to the teeth.

Dentists can provide fluoride treatment by administering concentrated fluoride gels or varnishes. Most gels use APF (acidulated phosphate fluoride), a formulation that allows teeth surfaces to quickly absorb it into their enamel layer: in fact, this happens within three to four minutes! Alternatively, your dentist may advise the application of a fluoride varnish, which usually comprises 5 per cent sodium fluoride.

Pit and Fissure Sealants

At the age of six, the first permanent molars make their appearance. The deep grooves on their chewing surfaces are surefire plaque traps. In order to seal them off from germ attack, your dentist may place 'pit and fissure sealants' (resins) into these grooves. It is ordinarily a quick, one-time procedure with minimal or no drilling, and they remain in place for years.

A bonus benefit of this treatment: through a totally painless procedure, it acclimatizes your child to the sound of the dental drill and the 'whoosh' of the suction tip draining out water from the mouth. It will surely ensure better cooperation from your child should he/she need more extensive treatment later.

Early Plaque Fighters

Children can develop gum problems too! Plaque accumulating on the teeth can solidify into tartar, leading to swelling or bleeding gums. At the dental clinic, the tartar can be gently cleaned away using ultrasonic instruments, in a procedure known as scaling. High-frequency sound waves, accompanied by a fine water spray clean the teeth thoroughly, and more importantly, *without any pain!*

Serial Extraction

At times, your dentist may detect a developing misalignment issue, especially if the milk teeth seem to be overstaying their welcome. In consultation with an orthodontist, he/she may recommend a procedure known as 'serial extraction', where such teeth are removed in a planned manner over a few months. This enables the permanent teeth to erupt into their designated positions, and thereby prevent major corrective treatment later.

Restoring Milk Teeth: Bring on the Kid Gloves

You now know of the far-reaching significance of milk teeth, and how imperative it is to preserve them in good health for their entire lifespan. Preventive measures go a long way in ensuring this. However, if these precautions have been inadequate, milk teeth can suffer damage, particularly through cavity formation. This would necessitate active treatment by your dentist to restore their health immediately, before it is too late to save them.

If your dentist can invest time and patience in managing children, they will cooperate fully with these procedures, at times even more so than adults! Many youngsters will allow the dentist to perform, often without any anaesthetic or under a local anaesthestic injection.

However, with children who are very young or mentally challenged or in the case of extremely uncooperative older children, the treatment may need to be carried out in a medical facility that supports the administration of general anaesthesia.

Your dentist is the best judge regarding use of any form of anaesthesia—whether to avoid it altogether or to use local or general anaesthetics.

Fillings, Endodontic Treatment and Extraction

Shallow cavities in milk teeth can be easily treated with fillings, and may be accomplished even without an anaesthetic. Some filling materials have an added benefit—they release fluoride!

For deeper cavities in milk teeth, the dentist's approach will depend on the child's age. In case it is close to the time of the tooth's shedding, the dentist may decide to extract it.

If a tooth decays much before its scheduled time of departure, a dentist could opt for endodontic treatment or root canal treatment to avoid extracting the tooth. For children, this could sometimes mean a partial root canal process called pulpotomy. After either of these procedures, the cleaned-out portion would need a strong filling. This may, or may not, be followed by a stainless steel crown or cap, which eventually falls off along with the milk tooth.

If the damage is too grave to restore, the tooth may need to be extracted well ahead of its time. In the case of a milk molar, your dentist will recommend a space maintainer—a small device fixed to the neighbouring tooth, which prevents infringement by other teeth. It will 'reserve' the space for the rightful permanent tooth, which will erupt at a later date. If this is not done, this space is lost and the permanent tooth might get crowded out, leading to misaligned teeth.

Orthodontic Treatment

Orthodontic treatment is best initiated in the early years, and the first visit to the orthodontist is recommended at around age seven. At this stage, he/she may be able to predict the way your child's teeth and jaws will develop and recommend corrective measures, if necessary.

This is also a good time for them to correct any undesirable habits, such as thumb-sucking or even mouth-breathing, as these can impact the alignment of teeth. Generally, most active orthodontic interventions for restructuring are performed between the age of eight and twelve. Chapter Seventeen discusses these in detail.

Mending Broken Teeth

The rough and tumble of childhood games occasionally results in broken teeth! Most routinely, an upper front tooth bears the impact, and suffers a 'fracture' or break.

If the broken piece of tooth can be found, please take it immediately to the dentist, who could try to bond it back into place. If the piece can't be found, and the break is not too close to the dental pulp, a skilled dentist can rebuild it with a cosmetic filling.

If the trauma to the tooth has breached the underlying pulp, an endodontic treatment might be carried out. Thereafter, the tooth is restored to its original size, shape and function, using cosmetic filling materials. Some teeth that are badly broken might even need a crown or cap in their reconstruction.

Rarely, an accident could result in total 'avulsion' of a permanent front tooth, wherein it is entirely pulled out of its bony socket in the jaw. If it can be found, please clean it gently to rinse off any grime. Please do not scrub it! The tooth can then be taken to the dentist either in a small container of cold milk, or even inside the child's mouth where the saliva can keep it protected.

If the dentist can see you within an hour, the chances of re-planting the tooth in its socket are high. He/she can stabilize the tooth by splinting it to its neighbouring teeth. If this procedure succeeds, the dentist may need to recommend an endodontic (root canal) procedure at a later date. Note, that this replanting option is not advisable in the case of a milk tooth that falls out due to injury.

Children's teeth play a vital part in their overall growth and development. Good parenting sets the stage for healthy dental habits, which will always stand your children in good stead. Their teeth are precious—please give them all the tender, loving care you can provide!

Chapter 7

Tooth Decay:
Stem the Mess

How does one even begin to understand a modern human disease that existed *before* humankind evolved? Tooth decay predates Homo sapiens, affecting even hominids like the Australopithecus. Ancient Indian, Roman, Sumerian and Chinese texts are full of evidence of the 'tooth worm' that caused the rot. In fact, even today, dentists in rural India are asked to remove and show the 'tooth worm' when patients visit their clinics!

Tooth decay is a global disease, and occupies a place in the top ten of health problems! Worldwide, while more than 80 per cent of the population is affected, only an insignificant percentile is aware of its causes or its prevention!

All about Tooth Decay: Know Thy Enemy

Well, so what is tooth decay, or dental caries as it is scientifically called?

It is an infection! Really! It took an inspired French surgeon and dentist, Pierre Fauchard, to look beyond the prayers to patroness Saint Apollina and to dismiss the 'worm' theory. Fauchard reasoned that bacterial activity in the mouth, along with sugar in our diet, was the primary cause of dental decay.

Simply put, an infection is the invasion of any body part by foreign organisms, which evade our defenses and then inflict damage to the structure. Some mouth bacteria gain a strong foothold on the teeth, and digest food residues lingering on them. This action releases powerful acids, causing damage to the hard tooth structure. The outcome: a hole or a cavity in the tooth!

An acquaintance with the enemy, and its strategies, is the first step in fighting the disease. So let's look closely at this germ attack to see how we can prepare against it.

To comprehend this complicated process, we must first acknowledge that our mouth is inherently a warehouse full of bacteria. There are good germs and bad germs, of which a few notorious ones like Streptococcus mutans, Streptococcus sobrinus and Lactobacillus cause the tooth to decay.

While we cannot see the bacteria, as they are microscopic, we can see plaque. Plaque is a thin, transparent or creamish film that easily sticks to the teeth surfaces. It teems with bacteria and is the biggest enemy of teeth and gums.

Plaque forms continually, even when we don't eat. This 'bio-film', with its superior glue-like feature, manages to adhere to all surfaces of the teeth.

Protected within this film lie a million bacteria, waiting for their fuel—fermentable carbohydrates, of which the most easily available is SUGAR! Whenever we eat starchy foods, our saliva starts digesting them to produce sugar.

Plaque bacteria love sugar. They consume it with glee, and as a by-product, produce strong acids. Some produce lactic acid, whereas others release pyruvic or formic acids. These are produced as quickly as within thirty minutes of us eating carbohydrates, with sugar-laden foods causing steep increase in acid levels in the mouth.

These acids gradually dissolve the hard armour of tooth enamel, in a process called demineralization. Furthermore, foods rich in acids like citrus fruits, colas and other aerated drinks add to and hasten, this degeneration. (Perhaps, that is why Pierre Fauchard advised mouth rinses with human urine as a remedy for tooth decay—urine's ammonia content would neutralize the acidity!)

Once the tooth enamel is breached, the bacteria can slowly continue their attack, destroying more of the tooth substance, and digging a hole in it!

Rough tooth surfaces favour the accumulation of plaque. This is one of the reasons why cavities are more commonly seen on the chewing surfaces of our molars, on which pits and grooves are inherently prevalent.

When plaque is not removed regularly, it also collects between adjacent teeth, causing decay on their contact surfaces. It is often surprising how cavities can occur in these parts, in the absence of decay on the chewing surfaces. The bitter truth is that food can stick to any surface of the tooth and so can plaque!

Thus, there are four factors necessary in the development of dental caries:

1. Plaque, which is full of harmful bacteria
2. Teeth with obvious or microscopic irregular surfaces for the plaque to cling to
3. Food that can be easily digested by the bacteria to release acids to demineralize the enamel
4. The duration for which the food is left on the teeth

The Stages of Tooth Decay: The Invader Marches On

In the initial stage, tooth decay might appear as a mere chalky-white area, where the early demineralization of tooth enamel has taken place. At this stage, cavities are painless, and can only be detected by a dentist. If the decay continues, it appears as a yellow, brown or black discolouration on the tooth. All cavities begin small, and more often than not—if left untreated—continue to rot at a slow pace, eventually becoming larger and delving deeper.

Stages of Tooth Decay

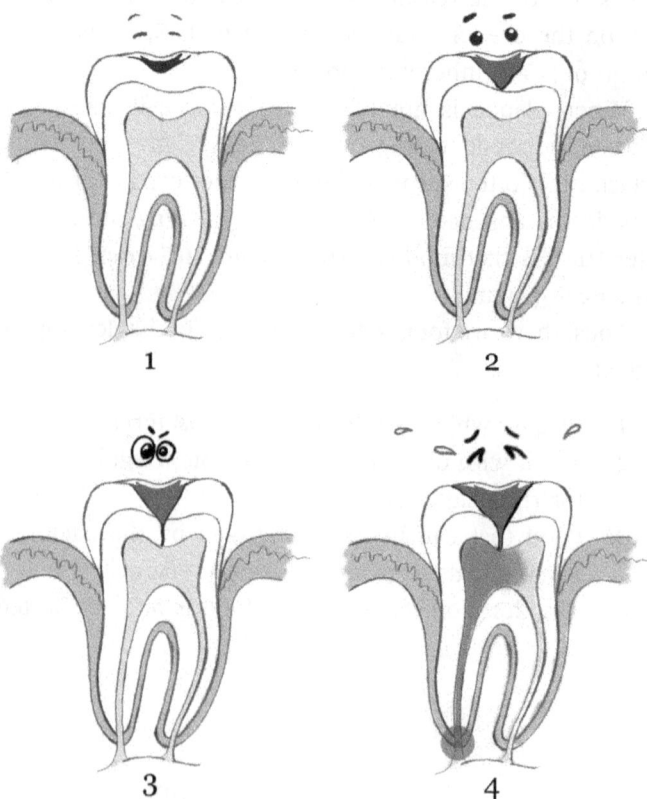

1

2

3

4

When the decay goes beyond the enamel to the underlying dentine, the cavities begin to look obvious, and since food particles tend to stick in them you could find yourself spending time after every meal wielding a toothpick! The classical sign of caries is the shock-like sensitivity experienced, albeit for a few seconds, when cold foods or sweets are consumed. Sufferers usually describe an odd sensation going right to their head. There's no pain yet.

As the cavity buries deeper into the tooth, the momentary response can turn into prolonged discomfort. One avoids eating on the affected side, as the tooth registers a sharp complaint. Of course, when the decay progresses and reaches the nerves in the core of the tooth—the pulp—the yelling-in-pain starts! The pulp tissue deteriorates, it loses its vitality and soon you have a dead tooth.

When the infection reaches even beyond the pulp and into the base of the root in the form of an abscess, then all hell breaks loose. The toothache can be so excruciating that your life can come to a standstill, often finding it difficult to even eat or sleep. If neglected, tooth infections can progress even further, leading to severe swellings inside and outside the mouth.

The Body Fights Back: Defence Ministry

Yes, our body has its defense mechanism to fight against this bacterial acid onslaught! Even as you read this, there is a cat-and-mouse game going on inside your mouth.

The frontline defense is our saliva. Apart from its primary purpose of lubricating food and kick-starting the digestive process, saliva also helps in protecting our teeth. Its flushing action clears food residues rapidly from the mouth, and its natural minerals help in reversing the demineralization of the enamel. Additionally, our saliva contains antibodies, which bind to bacteria and neutralize them.

The enamel, the outermost protective layer of the tooth is almost impervious to the acid; its primary mineral, hydroxyapatite, doesn't allow the acids to breach it easily. This layer is also constantly remineralised by the calcium salts in saliva.

Diagnosis of Dental Caries: On the Dentist's Chair

We often hear in our practice, 'Doctor, I never felt any pain. Do I really have cavities?' In the section above, you could see how cavities start to form, and then worsen progressively. The early stages are usually free of symptoms.

Therefore, dentists don't rely only on symptoms described by you, but look for telltale signs in the teeth. They use sharp instruments called probes or explorers, and sometimes bio-compatible dyes, to detect early or hidden cavities. X-rays, both analog and digital, and lasers are also useful tools for diagnosing the onset of cavities.

In deeper cavities, where the decay may have progressed into the pulp, the tooth can be under great pressure. Frequently, patients are unable to clearly point to the exact tooth that hurts, as the ache from that affected tooth can cause pain in the neighbouring ones, and to the underlying jaw as well. In such cases, the dentist might gently tap a few teeth in the area to discover the offending tooth.

Dentists use a universally accepted system for classifying tooth decay, based on its location. For example, decay can affect only the chewing surface of molar teeth (called a Class I cavity), or it may extend onto the surfaces where two adjacent teeth meet (called Class II cavities).

Diagnosing dental caries and its severity is best left to dentists, as subjective lay opinions can be thoroughly inaccurate! Unfortunately even today, grandparents, parents, aunts and uncles, co-workers, friends, neighbours and employees offer their views about teeth issues before one approaches the dentist!

Preventing Dental Caries: The Good Fight

Prevention is the best cure! Therefore, all measures should be taken to improve our oral hygiene, and reduce our tendency to eat easily fermentable carbohydrates like sugar.

Good oral hygiene practices are the key to keeping plaque off our teeth. Toothbrushing is a cardinal routine, and it is essential to brush twice daily. As salivary flow is restricted in sleep, brushing at night before going to bed is vital to ensure that these nocturnal bacteria do not have a free run.

If we minimize the exposure of our teeth to detrimental foodstuffs, we reduce the chances of caries. A nutritionally beneficial diet, deprived of fermentable carbohydrates like sugar, can go a long way in its prevention. The Chinese, with their reluctance for sweetened food, have the least number of people afflicted by tooth decay, while Indians are highly vulnerable to it due to our sugar-rich diet!

Rinsing the mouth well after eating is a great habit, as a good deal of food debris is washed away, starving the bacteria of their feasting. Finally, it is *vital* to floss your teeth at least once daily, reaching into the thin spaces between teeth where no brush stands a chance. By removing plaque from these areas, cavity formation can be prevented on such surfaces.

Treatment for Dental Caries: Charge and Attack!

The following questions are routinely thrown at dentists: 'Despite my best efforts, what if my tooth rots? What treatment options do I have?' Of course, it goes without saying that if attended to during the early stages, the procedures are less uncomfortable, less expensive and also require fewer visits to the dental clinic.

If the cavity is small, it is cleaned out, and a simple conservative filling is easily accomplished to restore the decayed portion of the tooth. If the cavity is deeper, extending into the sensitive dentine layer, but not yet affecting the pulp, a filling can still be done, with additional protective layers beneath it.

But, when the cavity has dug really deep and damaged the pulp, then the time for fillings is over!

Now, endodontic treatment (popularly known as root canal treatment or RCT) becomes necessary, followed up with a filling. A crown/cap is put in place for molars and premolars, and it is usually advised to protect these brittle load-bearing teeth from fracturing. The dentist will avoid crowns in the front teeth if the rot is not too extensive.

In the eventuality of the tooth being beyond redemption, where even endodontic treatment is untenable, then extraction is the only tragic option left to the dentist and patient.

A stitch in time saves nine—this couldn't be more true when it comes to cavities! It is prudent to avoid getting to a stage where we have to extract a tooth, for the tooth is meant to last our lifetime! Prevention and early intervention can turn the tide in our favour in the war against dental caries.

Chapter 8

Gum Disease:
Movers and Shakers

You eat right, exercise well and get your annual health checks done. All is well, right? Yet, chances are that you may still be suffering from the commonest disease in the world! Here's an astounding fact: 90 per cent of humans suffer from gum disease!

Gums: In Health

The gums are essentially the soft tissues that surround the neck of every tooth—essentially, the junction of the exposed and submerged parts of the tooth. The support system includes the gums, the jawbone and the periodontal ligament.

Healthy gums are usually light pink in colour, but this may vary by race, with degrees of dark pigmentation. Importantly, healthy gums do not bleed on touch, or while brushing and flossing the teeth. They feel firm, and remain in position, not allowing the roots of the teeth to be exposed.

Gums: In Sickness

The term 'gum disease' refers to conditions relating not just to the gums—it can affect the supporting jawbone and the

Gum Disease

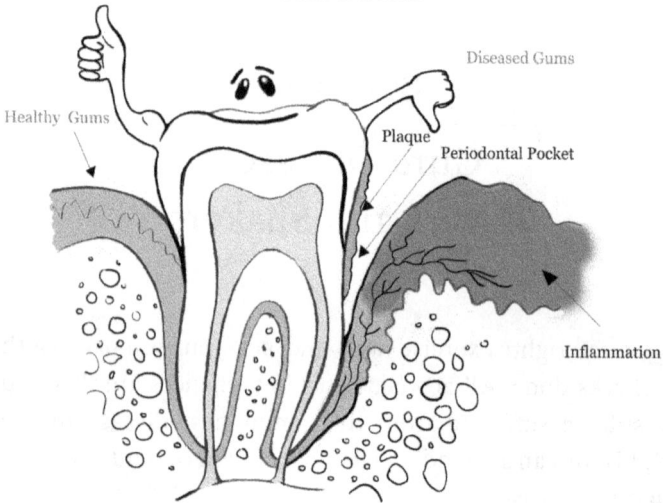

periodontal ligament too and hence, a more accurate term for this ailment would be 'periodontal disease'.

The early stage of gum disease is called gingivitis, which inflicts itself on nearly all of us to some degree. It is not an infection you catch—but is caused by the bacteria residing in your own dental plaque! They irritate the gum tissues by releasing toxic products, which cause the gums to swell up and bleed when you brush and floss, or even if you bite into firm foods. These are the typical symptoms. The gums also start looking more ruddy and may feel less firm; you may experience some bad breath too.

As more plaque accumulates, some of it starts to solidify into tartar. Once this hard tartar has formed, it cannot be cleaned away by a toothbrush or floss. Worse, the rough surface of tartar allows more plaque to build up. Strangely, there is usually no pain or discomfort associated with gingivitis—which explains why many sufferers ignore it!

Gingivitis is reversible: milder versions respond to home care, improving with better tooth brushing and flossing. If tartar has already formed, the dentist will remove it with a session of professional cleaning, in a procedure called scaling (more later!).

Gingivitis can persist for months or even years. If left untreated, it progresses to invoke damage to the deeper tooth-supporting structures. This condition is called periodontitis.

The tight connection between the gums and the teeth starts giving way, and the mouth bacteria begin to push into this area. The deeper zones, away from the surface, are low in oxygen content, favouring the growth of more destructive types of mouth germs called anaerobic bacteria. They merrily join the bandwagon and spur the ravaging of the supporting jawbone.

Our immune response launches a counter-attack, but some of the by-products of this inflammatory response also end up damaging other tissues (similar to the collateral damage during army operations). As supporting bone is lost, teeth start getting loose. This 'bone loss' can eventually lead to 'tooth loss'.

In the early stages, the symptoms are no different from those of gingivitis, namely, gums that are spongy or swollen, redder and bleeding. As the condition develops further, many new symptoms make an appearance:

- The gums begin to separate from the teeth, creating spaces between the two (these are called pockets).
- One may occasionally note a pus discharge from these pockets, especially when the gums are massaged. This had led to the old term, pyorrhea, for this condition (from *pyo*=pus; *-rrhea*=flow)
- Many complain of an itching in the gums, and bad

breath worsens.
- The mouth develops a 'bad' taste, and food flavours seem diminished.
- The gums tend to recede, and the teeth start looking longer.
- The teeth may move from their positions, and spaces open up between them.
- Some teeth can become very sensitive to cold or sweet foods, as the disease exposes their roots.
- Teeth feel loose, and the upper front teeth may protrude.
- As more teeth become loose, chewing becomes difficult, and the 'bite' position between your upper and lower teeth could change.
- Boils or abscesses can form within the gums, which may burst through the surface.
- In the final stages, the loosened teeth could actually fall right off.

Sadly, periodontal disease does not cause any pain till it has crossed the Rubicon, owing to which sufferers tend to seek help too late. Periodontitis is normally a slow, progressive disease, and most people who lose teeth to it are usually over the age of sixty.

There are more aggressive forms of this affliction, thankfully rare, which can cause severe damage and tooth loss in adolescents or young adults.

The Benefits of Healthy Gums: Treat 'em Right!

Keeping your gums healthy pays rich dividends! Here are the obvious benefits.

Your teeth stay strong, allowing you to chew all your favourite foods. (People with loose teeth often migrate towards softer high-calorie or high-fat foods, because they're easier to masticate and swallow, but are obviously less healthy.) Besides, your taste buds are sharper when gums are healthy—food seems more flavourful. And the roots of your teeth remain covered, allowing you to enjoy cold or sweet foods without any jolts of pain.

Healthy gums keep bad breath away, which can directly impact your social interactions. Moreover, oral hygiene becomes simpler—no gum bleeding and no unwieldy gaps between the teeth to manage! Healthy gums look good, and contribute immensely to the radiance of a smile.

There are some hidden, but very significant benefits to maintaining gum health! Alternatively, untreated gum disease can lead to other more serious illnesses.

Keeping your gums healthy lowers your risk of cardiovascular disease—recent research showing that gum disease *doubles* the risk of heart attacks and strokes! Some deadly gum-bacteria cause the release of toxic products into the blood, leading to thickening of heart vessels and of the carotid artery supplying blood to the brain. Thus, blood flow is restricted to both, the heart and brain, and predisposes to cardiovascular ailments. So go, grab that floss!

Diabetics are very prone to developing gum disease, but this can become a vicious cycle too: untreated gum disease itself causes an increase in blood sugar levels. Diabetics will find it easier to keep their sugar levels in check if they get treatment for their gum disease.

Gum disease in pregnancy can result in premature births or newborns with low birth-weight. Women who are planning a pregnancy would therefore do well to get their gums in order.

In people whose immunity is compromised—such as organ transplant recipients, cancer patients, those on steroids or those suffering from HIV—gum-disease bacteria can induce infections in other areas of the body, such as pneumonia. These can assume serious proportions, and a healthy mouth can help ward off these complications.

The Risk Factors for Gum Disease: Dangerous Business

The seriousness of gum disease varies from person to person, but there are some risk factors that can provoke it:

- Smoking decreases the immunity of the mouth, so smokers tend to have higher levels of periodontal disease. Also, the stains left behind by tobacco offer rough surfaces for plaque to thrive on.
- Some medications can interfere with gum health. Steroids reduce the immunity, and exacerbate gum disease. Gum disease can thrive in the large gum swellings caused by certain medications, such as those prescribed for controlling high blood pressure (Nifedipine, Amlodipine), for treating epilepsy (Phenytoin) or as immune-suppressants in transplant patients (Cyclosporine).
- Diabetes is strongly linked with increased periodontal disease—it affects the immune response, as well as the repair of gum tissues, making diabetics extremely prone.
- Stress foments silent warfare against your gums! It depresses your immunity, and you could become apathetic towards maintaining oral hygiene.
- Women using hormonal medication or oral

contraceptives tend to develop more severe forms of gum disease, as these medications boost the growth of some destructive mouth bacteria. For similar reasons, more incidences are seen during pregnancy and menstruation.

- Kids attaining puberty also suffer diseased and swollen gums, due to the sudden increase in hormones circulating in the blood.
- Your genetic makeup can decide your immunity to gum disease, or the intensity of your body's 'inflammatory response'. This may explain why people with similar oral hygiene standards and risk factors can end up with vastly different degrees of gum disease.

Preventing Gum Disease: Homing In

One of the most common myths is that your teeth will become loose and fall off when you get old. So, gum disease is inevitable, right? Wrong! The good news is that gum disease is *totally* preventable! You can, with the right measures, ensure that your gums remain healthy lifelong, and that you don't lose a single tooth even as you turn ninety!

The key to healthy gums is good home care, which boils down to proper toothbrushing, and flossing. Some people may need additional devices to clean between the teeth, the details of which you found in Chapter Three and which we explore further in Chapter Ten.

Let's highlight the significant weapons at your disposal to battle gum afflictions:

- Brushing your teeth twice daily, with a soft-to-medium toothbrush, which should be changed every two or three months

- Following the correct technique of brushing, with a gentle roll of the wrists
- Using fluoridated toothpaste whenever possible
- Flossing all the teeth at least *once a day*

There is really no need to use a finger to massage the gums. The act of toothbrushing itself provides a gum massage!

Apart from this, it also helps if you maintain a nutritious diet and keep off tobacco!

Battling Gum Disease: Doctor, Fix It!

Let your dentist participate in keeping your gums healthy! However well you perform your home dental care, the structure of our teeth is such that plaque and tartar still find their way into areas that are difficult to maintain.

Scaling

The simplest treatment for gum disease is professional cleaning of tartar deposition, known as scaling. Earlier, scaling was performed with manually operated instruments, known as hand scalers. These have sharp cutting edges, which scrape off the deposits from the teeth. While these are effective, the procedure is time consuming. Furthermore, the pressure needed to operate these instruments causes some discomfort to patients, and could also inflict scratches or gouges on the tooth roots.

Clinics now prefer the use of ultrasonic scalers to accomplish an efficient cleaning job. Here's the lowdown on them: these are electrically operated instruments, which use the energy of high-frequency sound waves to disrupt and disintegrate tartar deposits. The tips of these instruments are blunt, causing minimal or no discomfort. A fine mist of water is produced whenever the instrument is activated, which not only flushes away the debris, but also keeps the tip cool. They can be used on almost everyone, barring a few exceptions. (Some are not suitable for pacemaker-wearers, but safe variants are available.) Those with dental implants should inform their dentist, as they need special non-metallic tips to be used on them.

Dentists prefer to follow up on an ultrasonic scaling with a bit of manual scaling too, to achieve a good finish. Finally, a session of polishing, with an abrasive paste, cleans off the stains and rough surfaces produced by the scaling. The paste is rubbed over the teeth, using rotating dental drill tips that are like mini-brushes.

However, polishing, as a routine procedure, is now a debatable issue. There are concerns about the abrasion, and the thinning of tooth enamel, due to repeated applications. As modern ultrasonic scalers leave behind little or no staining or roughness, we prefer to restrict this procedure to exceptional cases.

Scaling eliminates tartar deposits, and the associated plaque. It allows the gums to get back to health, and all the symptoms of gingivitis are reversed. This practice is recommended at six-monthly intervals for all adults, towards maintaining healthy gums. As a bonus, the dentist gets to study all your teeth closely during the operation, leading to early detection of cavity formation or other abnormalities.

A common myth associated with scaling is that it causes the teeth to loosen. The truth is, scaling does exactly the opposite! It helps the gums to recover, and can actually help loose teeth firm up. The myth probably originated when scaling was done on teeth with severe loss of bone support, such teeth were perhaps being held together only by the cement-like tartar deposits! When the tartar went, the shakiness of the teeth would become apparent instantly, akin to that joke about an old battered car that is held together by the dirt on it!

Deep Cleaning

When gum disease progresses to the stage of periodontitis, further treatment becomes necessary. Early stages of this disorder can be managed conservatively, with 'non-surgical' procedures.

Your dentist may recommend a 'deep cleaning' under local anaesthesia. This is a combination of scaling, followed by 'root planing'—the gentle scraping of the surface of the tooth roots, which gets contaminated by deep tartar deposits and bacterial toxins. Dentists use fine instruments known as curettes to accomplish this, leaving the root surfaces clean and allowing gum health to be restored.

Depending on the severity, some antibiotics or antibacterial medication may be prescribed. Many benefit with this conservative therapy, and going forward, require nothing more than routine maintenance and scaling.

Surgical Procedures

When the gravity of periodontitis increases, it becomes difficult for the dentist to reach into the deep recesses under the gum line. At this stage, you may be referred to a periodontist, a specialist in gum diseases.

There are several types of surgical procedures that may be necessary to treat the disease. The commonest is periodontal flap surgery, causing very little discomfort and most people resume normal activities the very next day!

As part of this surgery, the affected area is first anaesthetized. The diseased gums are then gently peeled back off the teeth. This exposes the inner, damaged areas, which are thoroughly cleansed of damaged tissues, tartar and plaque deposits. The periodontist may occasionally place a substitute for the lost bone (known as a bone graft), and cover it with a thin film (known as a membrane), to allow lost bone to regenerate. The gums are then put back in place, and secured into position with stitches (sutures). The area heals up quickly, and the health of the gums improves tremendously.

Different surgeries may be necessary to correct various other gum problems too! Here are a few examples:

- Roots exposed due to gum disease can be covered by gum tissue from adjacent or even distant sections: this is known as grafting.
- People suffering from gum enlargement, usually as a result of medication, may require a procedure known as gingivectomy, where the excess gum tissue is trimmed away.
- On occasion, your dentist may suggest cutting back of gum tissue around teeth that need to be capped, known as crown lengthening.
- Muscle movement of the lip or tongue could sometimes pull at the gums, which would then need a process known as frenectomy to correct it.

Following most gum surgeries, painkillers are prescribed, and your dentist may recommend a course of antibiotics too. It is also advised to suspend toothbrushing and flossing in the operated area. Instead, a strong mouthwash, containing an antibacterial drug known as Chlorhexidine, is usually recommended for a few days, till normal oral hygiene practices can be resumed.

Long-term use of such mouthwashes is avoidable, as they leave side effects such as brown stains on the teeth, or even a loss of taste sensation.

The most common disease in the world starts innocuously enough, but can progress to a stage where teeth are lost—in fact, gum disease is the leading cause for this. Good home care and timely professional help can work wonders together to keep your gums in the pink of health, literally!

Chapter 9

Tooth Sensitivity:
Enjoy Your Ice Cream

The pleasure of having ice cream on a hot summer's day is an unparalleled one! Sadly, this can become a nightmare when one has sensitive teeth. Most people describe the sensation as a shock wave, travelling faster than the speed of lightning, from the teeth to the brain!

While *cold* is the most common trigger, various other stimuli can cause this too. Sweet and sour foods, or even a draught of air could spark the unpleasant feeling. The discomfort is usually brief, lasting a few seconds, but the sensation is acutely distressful. There are many who feel that it is easier to manage pain than to cope with the suddenness and intensity of *this* attack.

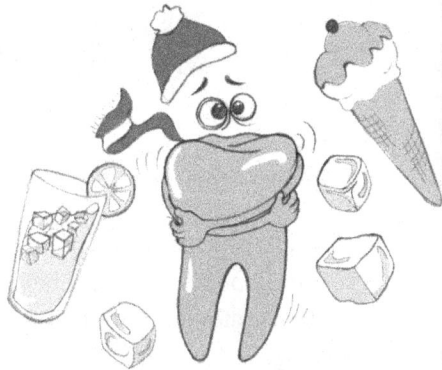

Dentinal Hypersensitivity: Having the Nerve

All teeth have some degree of thermal sensitivity—they feel the contact of very cold or hot foods, due to the nerves within the core of the tooth, the dental pulp. This is normal and doesn't cause hurt, as the pulp is well insulated by enamel, which is a protective shield around it. Healthy gums also cover the base of the teeth, preventing any sensations from contacting their roots, which are also protected by a softer material known as cementum.

When teeth become sensitive, it is because there is a breach or loss of these protective elements, which expose the next underlying layer, the dentin. Unlike enamel, which is insensitive, the dentine can conduct sensations to the pulp. Full of fine hollow tubes (dentinal tubules) of fluid, when food or liquids reach the dentin, the fluid in these tubules gets agitated. This disturbance sends a response to the nerves present in the pulp and stimulates acute pain. Dentists call this condition 'dentinal hypersensitivity'.

Triggers of Dentinal Hypersensitivity: A Delicate Matter

Cavities, especially in the early stages, can cause pain that mimics hypersensitivity. They, too, expose the dentin, making the tooth momentarily reactive, especially to cold foods and beverages. As cavities burrow deeper, this ache persists for a longer period. Similar pain also results from leaky fillings and crowns.

Hypersensitivity can occur due to a variety of reasons.

Gum Recession

The commonest cause of hypersensitivity is gum recession, which exposes the cementum protecting the roots of the teeth, and which soon wears away. The dentin underneath gets uncovered and leads to the sensitivity.

Gum recession has two main causes:

- Incorrect toothbrushing: Horizontal strokes of the brush cause injury to the gums. The gums recede, exposing the roots to the abrasive forces of the brush. Hard toothbrushes and grainy powders used for cleaning the teeth in many countries, produce similar results.
- Gum disease: When simple inflammation of the gums or gingivitis is left untreated, the disease progresses to the deeper recesses of the gums. The bone supporting the teeth gets damaged and makes the gums recede.

Tooth Wear and Tear

Wearing away of the tooth surface is another major contributor to hypersensitivity. This happens in many ways:

- Thinning of enamel from the chewing surfaces (known as attrition), due to tooth-grinding habits
- Severe attrition due to habits such as chewing paan, betel nut, etc., or/and prolonged use of chewing gum
- Using rough tooth powders to clean the teeth, including coarse salt, burnt rice husk, among others
- Use of hard toothbrushes

Enamel Erosion

Tooth enamel can suffer erosion—it dissolves due to chemical insult. This bares the dentin, causing hypersensitivity, and can happen in a variety of ways.

For instance, during pregnancy, many women suffer from nausea and vomiting. The stomach acids in the vomit cause the enamel to dissolve.

Moreover, people who tend to keep multiple fasts could invite increased acidity. The unused digestive acids may travel up to the mouth and cause erosion of the teeth. A similar problem occurs in those with a stomach-reflux disorder.

Besides, habits like excessive consumption of aerated drinks, acidic food, sucking of lime, etc. can also erode the enamel. Children, especially teenagers, are heavy consumers of cold, carbonated drinks that cause sensitivity.

Dental Procedures

During the whitening of teeth, both at the dental clinic and with home-based products, some tooth sensitivity could ensue. The active chemical ingredients in the bleach penetrate the enamel, and work on lightening the colour of the underlying dentin. The dentin suffers mild irritation, causing the transient pain.

Teeth may become sensitive following certain dental treatment procedures:

- Fillings that are deep may cause irritation to the pulp.
- If a filling has a 'high' spot, a raised portion that alone contacts the opposing tooth, it can come under pressure and turn sore.
- Teeth are shaped down to accommodate crowns and bridges—this removes most of the enamel, exposing the dentin, and if a temporary crown or bridge is not placed immediately, these teeth can be at a high risk of torment.
- Post-scaling, teeth can experience sensitivity if the roots that were covered by tartar deposition are exposed.
- Following the application of orthodontic braces, due to the increased pressure on the teeth.

Chipped and Broken Teeth

Teeth that suffer injury may get chipped or broken, exposing the sensitive dentin. Some teeth develop cracks, extending deep into the core and become hypersensitive.

At the Dentist's for Dentinal Hypersensitivity: Professional TLC

While tooth sensitivity is not as debilitating as pain from tooth decay, it can be agonizing when it occurs. We need to understand that this sensation is only a symptom, and its treatment lies in correcting the actual cause of the condition. More often than not, the dentist is not approached when the discomfort begins, but much later.

Your dentist can help nip the problem in the bud by diagnosing and treating the underlying cause.

In the case of a cavity or a leaky restoration, he can address this with the appropriate treatment. In deep cavities, dentists will shield the pulp using a protective layer known as a liner, under the filling.

Similarly, chipped or cracked teeth need to be fixed to prevent them from reacting. If a filled tooth or a replacement is 'high'—in other words, coming into undue contact with the opposing tooth—the chewing surface will be adjusted to avoid the sensitivity.

When gum disease is present, teeth can be professionally cleaned to eliminate plaque and tartar. Additional treatment may be necessary in case of severe gum affliction.

When teeth are prepared for crowns and bridges, they can be coated with protective sealants to prevent leakages, and to reduce immediate post-procedural soreness.

Areas, where tooth substance (enamel or cementum) has worn off, would need fillings to restore the lost structure, and to stem the vulnerability.

If there is excessive tooth wear due to a tooth-grinding

habit, the dentist can provide a preventive device known as a night-guard.

If the tenderness is due to a minor abrasion of the tooth substance, a conservative approach to treatment is favoured— your dentist may advise the use of a de-sensitizing toothpaste and mouthwash. The commonly used active ingredients, strontium and fluoride, work on the principle of blocking the dentinal tubules, so that they don't transmit sensations to the nerves in the pulp. Another ingredient—potassium nitrate—numbs the tooth nerve to prevent feeling.

Recent introductions, which also rapidly block the dentinal tubules, include a combination of calcium carbonate and arginine, or calcium sodium phosphosilicate (a bioactive glass). Anti-cavity tooth crèmes or dental mousses have a numbing effect as well. They contain a milk derivative called casein phosphopeptide combined with amorphous calcium phosphate (a proprietary preparation called Recaldent™).

The use of these desensitizing formulations is advocated *only* after the dentist ascertains that the cause of pain doesn't need other corrective measures. They take effect in a few days, though some of the newer compounds promise instant relief.

Desensitizing toothpastes may be used in one of several ways:

- To replace your normal toothpaste, and brush twice daily with it
- To apply on the teeth for a few minutes before brushing it off
- To apply a thin film of paste on your teeth just before retiring at night

Desensitizing mouthwashes contain potassium nitrate, usually combined with fluoride. These should to be used undiluted, rinsing for at least a minute before spitting out. Ideally, it's best to avoid food or drink for twenty to thirty minutes after this, and to avoid rinsing with water immediately after.

Self-care for Dentinal Hypersensitivity: You Can Help

Some of the reasons for tooth sensitivity can be addressed at home; here's what you can do:

Brush Right

Brushing too hard, or using vigorous horizontal strokes injure the gums and wear away the tooth enamel. Brush with a gentle rolling of the wrists, with a soft or medium toothbrush. Use toothpastes, not abrasive powders!

Cut the Cola

Erosion of teeth that occurs because of aerated drinks can be easily avoided by reducing their excessive consumption.

Shed the Chewing Habit

Teeth surfaces can get severely thinned down if you have a chewing habit, be it paan or tobacco. This makes them extremely sensitive, and can even wear down enough to expose the nerves in the tooth.

Stop Gnashing

You can address attrition of teeth and loss of enamel due to grinding by becoming aware of the habit, and consciously avoiding it. If you've been advised wearing a night guard, please do so!

Keep Gums in the Pink of Health

Keep your gums healthy! Don't allow them to recede and open the gates to sensitivity. Brush and floss daily, and get regular professional cleaning done to help ward off gum disease.

Beware of the Acid

Frequent vomiting can cause enamel to erode. As vomiting during pregnancy is common, expectant mothers must take care to rinse their mouth clean of any acidic residue after the bouts of sickness. Avoid indulging in habits like sucking on lime—your enamel can melt away!

We love eating and drinking a wide range of food and drink. We relish our ice cream, a hot cuppa or a chilled beer too! We can continue to enjoy these simple pleasures of life, only if our teeth approve! Timely professional attention and good home care can keep tooth sensitivity at bay. Cheers!

Chapter 10

Bad Breath:
Fume and Fret

In India, it is considered respectful to offer a guest paan after a meal. Paan is a betel leaf, in which additives like betel nut, lime and often tobacco are stuffed. This is chewed for its purported properties as a digestive, mouth freshener and a carminative. Some versions also contain flavouring ingredients such as aniseed, cardamom, etc.

One of the main reasons for chewing paan is that it masks mouth odours—your guests can enjoy your hospitality without reciprocating with their bad breath! Various cultures had their own equivalents for freshening the mouth—Italians preferred chewing parsley and ancient Chinese texts recommended ground eggshells. In fact, bad breath or halitosis had been mentioned since ages past; it was even a major concern for the Pharaohs! Of course, the ancient Egyptians also had a remedy—tablets containing a concoction of myrrh, cinnamon and honey!

More recently, in the early part of the twentieth century, a surgical antiseptic and floor cleaner was reformulated, and this lowly disinfectant morphed into the first modern mouthwash! It is an alcohol-based solution, and is still hugely popular, thus bringing halitosis out of the closet. In fact, its marketing focused on the importance of clean breath in finding a marriage partner, projecting halitosis as a serious obstacle. Not a new idea at all though—in the ancient Jewish world, marriages could be annulled on these grounds!

Halitosis: Smelling a Rat

The word halitosis is a combination of two terms: the Latin 'halitus' (breath) and the Greek '-osis' (pertaining to disease/condition); bad breath is also known as 'oral malodour'. More than 90 per cent of the offensive smell originates from the mouth, while the rest is related to other causes.

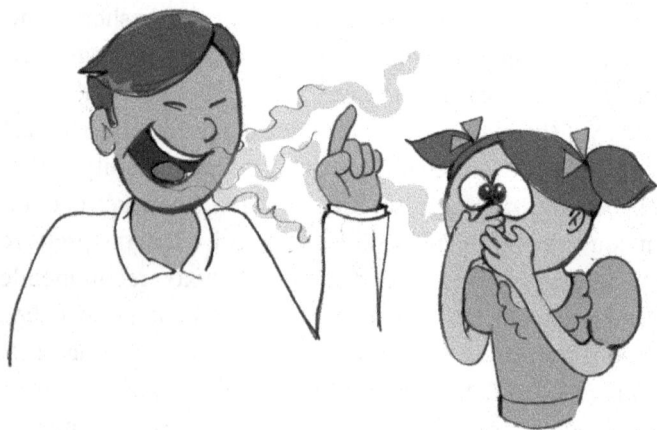

The Mouth and Anaerobes: Foul-mouthed?

The mouth is home to more than 600 different kinds of bacteria! Most of these are harmless and don't have any strong links with bad breath. Several, however, are anaerobes, which means that they can go about their business without oxygen. When these bacteria get an opportunity to thrive, they set up a putrefaction process, whose by-products are formidably foul smelling.

Protein is available to these bacteria from residual food particles in the mouth, especially fish, meat and dairy, or vegetable sources like onions and garlic, and even from saliva. They cause these residues to rot, releasing smelly substances known as volatile sulphur compounds (VSC). One VSC, hydrogen sulphide, smells of rotten eggs, while another, methyl mercaptan, of a gas leak. Other smelly villains, the 'indigoids' such as indole and skatole, also lend their distinctive odour to faeces! Bacteria also produce compounds known as polyamines, such as putresceine and cadaverine (the terms are kind of self-explanatory!).

Where Anaerobes Thrive: Not Smelling of Roses

There are a few main areas in the mouth where these anaerobes thrive.

The Rear Portion of the Tongue

In what could come as a surprise to most people, the key source of bad breath is at the back of the tongue! The tongue's surface is naturally uneven, and provides an opportunity for bacterial buildup. Added to this are layers of dead cells from the mouth lining, as well as food debris. The resultant coating is a potent recipe for halitosis. As the roughness of the tongue surface varies from person to person, so does the tendency for bad breath.

Gum Pockets Found in Gum Disease (Periodontitis)

Periodontitis is a severe form of gum disease, where deep crevices called pockets, form between the teeth and the gums.

These pockets harbour masses of anaerobic bacteria, which can cause severe halitosis.

Undisturbed Dental Plaque on the Teeth

Dental plaque formation on teeth surfaces is a continuous process because of bacterial accumulation, due to poor oral hygiene habits. While most people brush their teeth regularly, they forget to floss. As a result, plaque remains fixed between the teeth, allowing growth of anaerobic bacteria. Physically and mentally challenged people could also find it tough to maintain good oral hygiene, predisposing them to halitosis.

Miscellaneous Spots in the Mouth

Apart from these major areas, there are umpteen others:

- Wounds in the mouth that can exist due to tooth extraction, mouth ulceration, surgery, etc., all of which prevent normal oral hygiene practices and allow plaque and food debris to accumulate
- Decaying teeth, which trap food debris and foster further rot
- Unclean dentures, as quite a few wearers don't keep their dentures clean—loads of plaque and food can come to stay, especially on the fitting surfaces, and cause bad breath
- Leaky fillings or crowns, which are traps for food debris and bacteria

Beyond the Mouth

A small number of causes for halitosis—less than 10 per cent—can be found away from the mouth:

- Nose: Infections in the nose, particularly sinusitis, can

result in bad breath. Sinusitis leads to a post-nasal drip, which could leave residues at the back of the tongue.

- Throat: Infection of any of the tonsils (protective glands found in the throat) can give rise to bad breath.
- Lungs: Infections like pneumonia and bronchitis can create a malodorous mouth.
- Hormonal conditions: Women can suffer from halitosis during menstruation and ovulation, or if they are taking oral contraceptive pills.
- Indigestion: Belching and acid reflux from the stomach can exude bad smells from the mouth.
- Diabetes mellitus: Patients whose glucose levels are very high may develop breath that smells of nail-polish remover (acetone breath). They are also prone to developing fungus infection in the oral cavity.
- Kidney disease: Renal impairment or failure causes increased of toxic urea in the body, leading to a 'fishy' or 'ammonia-like' breath.
- Liver failure: Multifarious toxins can amass in the blood if the liver is incapacitated, leading to a foul musty breath (called foetor hepaticus).

Causes of Halitosis: Smelling Fishy

Apart from anaerobes, there are several other causes for bad breath:

- Smoking, which apart from an unpleasant smell, also leaves behind a dry mouth and possible gum disease, both predisposing to halitosis
- Ingesting smelly foods like onions, garlic, cabbage, cauliflower, radish, etc., which allow bacteria to work

    on them and release VSCs
- Consuming alcohol, which is very much like smelly foods—in that it continues to emit odour later, too (through exhaled breath, as a result of by-products from our own digestive processes)

Local remedies to mask such odours may be useless. Till the smells are completely expelled by the lungs, the breath will continue to smell foul.

There is another oft-forgotten reason for bad breath: mouth dryness. Without the protective flow of saliva, bacteria in the mouth grow rapidly, and release their stinky qualities. There are several causes of mouth dryness:

- Fasting (which leads to 'hunger breath')
- Mouth-breathing habit
- Smoking
- Alcohol consumption
- Mouthwashes containing alcohol (it is indeed ironic that the very product used commonly to avoid halitosis can actually aggravate the issue!)
- Salivary gland dysfunction, as any disease or condition affecting the functioning of salivary glands may lead to decreased flow of saliva
- Medications, especially some drugs that cause mouth dryness as a side effect, including medication for hypertension, depression and allergies—Sildenafil, too, please note!

Diagnosis of Halitosis: Sniffing It Out

So, how would you know if you have bad breath? It seems fairly straightforward: breathe out through the mouth into a cupped hand and sniff to check, yes? Well, not really! One of the unfortunate things about halitosis is that plenty of victims are unaware of the condition—their noses may be acclimatized to their stinking mouths, and so fail to detect the 'dragon breath'!

Therefore, people rely on asking a friend about whether their breath smells bad or not, and this could be a fairly accurate gauge (you may lose a friend, though!).

Suggestions to diagnose one's own bad breath have been around for a while. One advises you to lick the back of your hand, and take a whiff. Another one is to scrape the back of your tongue with a spoon and sniff the stuff. Of course, these are subjective, and you could take the results with a pinch of (smelling?) salt.

At the professional level, numerous dental clinics have equipment to detect halitosis. One of these measures the level of VSCs in the breath. Other tests require sending a breath sample to a lab for testing, where a gas chromatograph reads out the results. Labs can also test samples of saliva to check for specific bacteria and their noxious spinoffs.

Preventing Halitosis: Slay the Dragon!

To prevent (or even fight!) halitosis, here is what *you* can do:

Aim for a Clean Mouth

Good oral hygiene is the cornerstone of your battle against bad breath. Needless to say, brushing your teeth twice daily and flossing them at least once are the bare minimum requirements.

Brushing in the morning helps rid the accrual of nocturnal

plaque and bacteria, and so freshens the breath. The unpleasant 'morning breath' can be compounded by a mouth-breathing habit too.

Brushing at night is crucial, as the mouth dries up while you sleep owing to reduced salivary flow, allowing increased bacterial growth.

Flossing and other interdental aids, dislodge bacteria from between the teeth—areas which cannot be reached by a toothbrush.

To prevent halitosis, the most important part of the oral hygiene regimen is to clean the tongue! As more than 80 per cent of bad breath originates from its surface, a good tongue cleaning process can ensure long-lasting fresh breath.

The best way to clean the tongue is to scrape away the coating formed on its surface. Plastic scrapers are ideal, as chances of injury are avoided. Some scrapers are designed with an uneven edge to adapt better to the rough texture of the tongue. It may be worth getting your hands on one.

Tongue scrapers work well with firm pressure, but too much force can cause bleeding or cuts! They need to reach as far back on the tongue as possible. Initially, this may cause a gagging sensation, but it settles with time; if the tongue is kept stiff during the cleaning, the chances of that sensation are reduced.

A toothbrush can also step in to sweep over the tongue surface, but may not be as effective as a scraper.

Oral irrigators, which use a forced jet of water, can flush away food debris and loose plaque, and are particularly useful in people undergoing orthodontic treatment.

Rinsing the mouth well after meals flushes away food debris, and goes a long way in preventing bad breath.

Eat on Time

Eat meals on time, and avoid long hours of fasting. If you cannot eat, sip water or fluids frequently to keep the mouth hydrated.

Shun Smelly Foods When You Have To

Especially before social engagements, avoid eating foods like onion, garlic, fish and radish, which not only taint the mouth, but also cause a lingering breath malodour over a few hours. People may avoid you!

Avoid Smoking and Tobacco

Smoking has manifold ill effects, ranging from gum disease to cardiovascular disorders, mouth cancer and bad breath too!

Avoid all forms of chewable tobacco, as it stains the teeth, allowing plaque and tartar to collect. Tobacco also aggravates gum disease, setting the grounds for bad breath.

Say No to Liquor

Restrict alcohol consumption, as it dries the mouth, promoting bad breath. The reek of exhaled alcoholic breath is pretty disgusting, you'd agree!

Scrub Those Dentures

If you wear removable dentures, ensure that they are kept scrupulously clean. If left dirty, they become slimy, and can irritate the gums and other mouth tissues as well.

Love Your Mouthwash, but with Discretion

Here's an important one: avoid those that contain alcohol! A variety of such commercially available mouthwashes cause a rebound dryness of mouth. Though they may give you a false sense of freshness, they can actually aggravate halitosis.

Every mouthwash has a bactericidal action; in other words, mouthwashes kill all the mouth bacteria. But, this can upset the equilibrium between the beneficial and harmful bacteria; the baddies often develop resistance, and tend to thrive more vigorously than the poor virtuous ones.

Also, prolonged use of mouthwashes could stain the teeth, providing the right surface for bacteria to prosper. We believe that mouthwashes could be used occasionally, but not over the long-term.

Chew Away

Chewing gum can help! Flavoured, sugar-free gum chewed over short durations (lest it stresses the joint between the upper and lower jaws) is effective in reducing bad mouth odours. It promotes salivation, which in turn combats halitosis, and has some cleansing effect on the teeth to boot.

Home Remedies for Halitosis: Granny Finale

Traditional home remedies for bad breath are as old as bad breath itself! A number of these relied on the belief that indigestion and stomach gases are responsible for this malady. As a result, many of grandma's stomach medicines have been used to cure it! In fact, a concoction called 'mukhwaas' ('mukh' is mouth; 'waas' is smell) is routinely eaten after meals in India, both to freshen the breath and to aid digestion. This is a mix of fennel, anise, caraway and sesame seeds, with some mint flavouring thrown in.

Meswak twigs (similar to the datun twigs used in India) popular in the Middle-East, are chewed to boost salivation, and for their cleansing action on teeth. Spices like cardamom and cloves can lend their delectable aromas to breath and are favoured in the East, while parsley leaves and peppermint are promoted in the West. Homemade mouth rinses could contain a decoction of either Eucalyptus leaves, or tea-tree oil, or baking soda. Even a dash of urine has been tried as an antidote to bad breath!

Unfortunately, most of these remedies focus on masking mouth odour and don't address the root causes. Obviously, the results offer only a temporary reprieve for sufferers, and for the people around!

Battling Halitosis at the Dentist's: Doctor Nose Best!

While the emphasis on preventing bad breath is on self-help, dentists can create favourable conditions to aid your efforts. The following treatments from your dentist will help:

- A professional cleansing of the teeth, to eliminate tartar deposits and associated plaque collection
- Repairing cracked or broken fillings, and correcting leaky crowns or bridges
- Filling deep cavities, which allow food particles to collect and stagnate
- Treating gum disease, and eliminating gum pockets which can foster anaerobic bacteria
- Treating oral infections, wounds or ulcers that can lead to halitosis
- Demonstrating oral hygiene techniques that will help prevent foul breath

Bad breath can be a huge social liability, but can also indicate the existence of more serious dental or medical conditions.

Patients need to see a dentist without delay, for diagnosis and solutions to eliminate the problem. If the cause is not connected with the mouth, dentists will guide their patients to a physician or the correct specialist, who can then address the underlying issue and control the malodour.

Simple home care goes a long way in preventing halitosis, so this is the time to grab that toothbrush!

Chapter 11

Bruxism:
Back to the Grind

Grinding and gnashing of teeth (bruxism) is a common human reaction, brought about by anger, resentment, and any other form of emotional distress. This is not a modern problem, for a verse in the Bible (Luke 13:28) mentions that 'there will be weeping [...] and gnashing of teeth...' when you find yourself excluded from the kingdom of God.

The term 'bruxism' refers to the abnormal and forceful clenching of the teeth. We all use our teeth to grind down our food, but here's an interesting fact: all meals put together, we chew for a sum total of not more than thirty to forty-five minutes in a day!

For the rest of the time, the upper and lower teeth keep a distance between each other, known as 'freeway space'. This position is maintained by the resting state of the jaw muscles, and is necessary in avoiding the contact of our

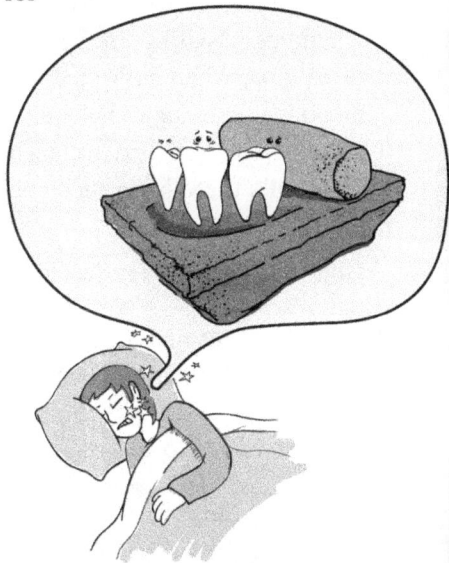

upper and lower teeth when not required. You will perhaps remember that our tooth enamel is a precious, non-renewable substance—it is designed to last a lifetime, provided we use it only for its intended functional role of biting and chewing!

Sleep and Awake Bruxism: Night and Day

Bruxism occurs more commonly in sleep (known as sleep bruxism), and less often in the daytime (known as awake bruxism).

In sleep bruxism, most sufferers are unaware of the habit until the person sleeping nearby tells them about the gnashing sound! Night bruxism is usually a combination of the grinding and clenching of teeth. This can continue for several minutes intermittently and generally happens during the stages of sleep arousal, when there is a change from deep sleep to lighter sleep.

During awake bruxism, there is normally more of teeth clenching and only the occasional grinding, but the person continues to remain unaware of the habit. It occurs more when engrossed in an activity, like working at the computer or driving, when subjected to boredom (such as attending a meeting) or being reprimanded.

More women tend to clench or gnash their teeth during the day, while there is no such gender bias among sleep bruxers.

High Risk Age Categories: The Era of Grinding

Bruxism is termed a parafunctional activity, as it is outside of the actual functioning ambit of the teeth. This habit is not restricted to grownups, but affects kids too!

It is easier to diagnose in children, as parents are often

awake when they sleep, and can recognize the sound of teeth gnashing when it happens. Traditionally, bruxism in children was attributed to worms in the tummy and grandma's recipes for deworming were followed. While there is no harm in deworming children on a regular basis, parents will realize that despite the medication, the bruxism doesn't cease.

In adults, this ailment affects all age groups, though there are indications that it happens much less in those over sixty. Studies reveal that bruxism affects nearly 20 per cent of the population, but this figure may actually be much higher, as the condition is not easy to discover.

Causes of Bruxism: Grounds for Grinding

A clear-cut cause for bruxism has still not been identified, but there are many suspects.

Psychological Stress

The prime suspect, especially in awake bruxing, it is relatively easy to identify the correlation between psychological tension and teeth grinding. Most of us are stressed in our daily routine, and fail to realize that such stress is cumulative. The hectic pace of modern-day living is a prescription for pent-up emotions and frustrations. Bruxism is the body's attempt to release the neuromuscular tension that accrues.

Children, too, are under tremendous pressure in their tender minds, and are often unable to cope with the increased strain of school, tests and parental expectations. This can manifest as bruxism.

Disturbances in Brain Chemicals

The brain is the powerhouse of our nervous system, and

controls all the muscular activity of our jaws, facial muscles and some muscles of the neck as well. Chemicals in the brain called neurotransmitters, regulate its system of producing electrical signals.

Bruxism has been seen to be associated with disturbances in one of these neurotransmitters known as dopamine. This could cause repetitive muscular contractions and rhythmic clamping of the jaw. The reasons for the disturbance are yet unknown, but there are indications that psychological tension may activate it.

Dental Causes

Misaligned teeth have been implicated in causing bruxism, as an attempt by the jaws to self-regulate the occlusion (the meeting of upper and lower teeth). Lots of people with mal-occlusion stress the temporomandibular joint—the paired ball-and-socket joint connecting the jaws, and located just in front of the ears. Similarly, ill-adjusted fillings or artificial teeth may force one to clamp hard in an attempt to set the 'bite' right.

Heredity

One theory states that there could be an inherent tendency for bruxism; some studies have concluded that children of parents who suffer from bruxism are more likely to become victims themselves.

Alterations in Dopamine Levels

Since the neurotransmitter dopamine has been associated with bruxism, changes in the dopamine level are likely to precipitate the condition.

Smokers are known to have a higher likelihood of bruxism—due to nicotine in the cigarette, which stimulates the brain to release more dopamine.

Also, drugs—in both prescribed and abused conditions—alter the dopamine levels and can cause the condition. For instance, Ecstasy users are known to brux their teeth. Patients with Parkinsonism on long-term medication to alter their dopamine levels, also show more instances of this problem. Many drugs for psychiatric illnesses, like bipolar disorder, could also similarly stimulate bruxism. Children on medication for attention deficit disorders also exhibit an increased tendency to it.

Symptoms of Bruxism: Ground Zero

Bruxism affects a significant percentage of the population, but is yet a tricky customer—most sufferers are not only unaware of its existence, but are actually in strong denial of the fact!

However, it always leaves behind several clues to its presence, and here are some of the symptoms *you* can watch out for.

Headache

While there are many causes for headache, the one associated with bruxism is typically experienced upon waking up. Some of the muscles involved in chewing are also connected to the scalp, neck and back muscles, and all these feel sore. Typically, you would complain of a dull headache especially in the morning, which dissipates as the day progresses.

Restless Sleep

Sufferers, characteristically, feel that their sleep was not restful, as they would have spent several hours through the night clenching and grinding.

Earache

Many bruxers complain of earache and land up visiting the ENT surgeon! In due course, they are referred to the dentist for a consultation. The pain actually originates in the temporomandibular joint. This joint comes under tremendous pressure, and gets inflamed due to the excessive force applied during bruxism. In some instances, it also develops into the painful condition of arthritis, undergoing irreversible damage with hastened wear and tear.

Pain in the Jaws

If you suffer from awake bruxism, there could be constant pain in the jaws through the day, due to straining of the jaw muscles.

Difficulty Opening the Mouth

The soreness affecting the temporomandibular joint and the jaw muscles, leads to trouble in opening and closing the mouth.

Joint Noise

Some bruxers can hear clicking or popping sounds from the temporomandibular joint, especially when opening the mouth wide or yawning. Often, the person sleeping next to you notices the grinding noises when you are asleep.

Dental Symptoms

Bruxism causes exaggerated wearing away of the chewing surfaces of all the teeth—this attrition leads to generalized hypersensitivity in many of them.

You would probably feel that your teeth turn sharp, and you could develop an ache in the tongue, inner cheeks and lips, as they all come between the teeth during the act of bruxism.

You could hurt while chewing food, at times even soft food. Moreover, your teeth could feel loose, caused by the excessive pressure on the periodontal ligament supporting them.

Signs of Bruxism at the Dentist's: Grist for the Mill

Dentists can recognize the signs of bruxism during routine examinations, and apprise you of the presence of this insidious habit. Here's what the dentist will check for:

- Sharp edges of the teeth
- Accelerated wear on the chewing surfaces of the teeth, not commensurate with your age
- Notched, chipped or fractured teeth
- Teeth that are shaky or 'mobile', in the absence of gum disease
- Generalized hypersensitive response from all the teeth to a blast of cold air
- Wearing away of the enamel along the necks of the teeth
- Clicking sounds, or pain in the temporomandibular joint when you open and close your mouth
- Loss or thinning of contact areas between teeth
- Indentations in the tongue, which tends to get bitten during bruxing
- Signs of repeated inner-cheek bites
- Repeated breakage of fillings, or dislodgement of crowns/bridges or implants
- Increase in size of the masseter muscle—extending from the area in front of the ear, till the angle of the jaw—one of the most used in grinding and clenching
- An altered shape to the face—squarer and firm—due to overuse of the masseter muscle

Combating Bruxism: You're Grounded!

Bruxism is a shadowy disease—sufferers deny it, and there is usually no clearly discernible cause. The commonest approach, therefore, is directed towards mitigating the damage done to the teeth and the temporomandibular joint.

Treatment of Obvious Dental Repercussions

Fillings, dentures or crowns that are out of alignment are corrected. Sharp teeth need to be rounded out. New fillings, crowns and veneers may have to be made for the worn out teeth to restore both function and aesthetics, and to correct any hypersensitivity.

Bite Guards

The technical name for such a guard is an 'occlusal splint'. Acting as shock absorbers, they prevent the upper and lower teeth from meeting each other, thus preventing the surfaces from wearing away. They are designed to be worn at night, and custom-made to fit snugly on your teeth in any one jaw only. But they could be ineffective in stopping the clenching and clamping associated with bruxism.

These guards are fabricated in a dental laboratory using a replica of your teeth, while some versions can be customized and fitted on in the clinic itself. Some are made of a hard acrylic material, while others are formed from softer vinyl. Since they are translucent, they could even be used during the daytime whenever feasible

A newer addition to the range of occlusal splints is a device known as an NTI-TSS (nociceptive trigeminal inhibition–tension suppression system). This is a customized partial splint—it covers only two to four upper front teeth. Made of rigid material, it blocks all contact between the upper and lower chewing teeth. It totally eliminates tooth grinding, clenching and clamping, since it is not possible to exert any appreciable clenching force with our front teeth.

Worn at bedtime and removed upon waking up, its daytime use may be difficult, as it is a bit of an eyesore—like a big bump under the upper lip. Yet, a spin-off of this concept can be useful for awake bruxers: they could try keeping the tip of the tongue between the upper and lower front teeth if they realize that they are tending to clench. This relaxes the jaw muscles and arrests daytime clenching.

Medication

A wide variety of drugs have been tried out in treating bruxism, including muscle relaxants, anti-anxiety medications, and anticonvulsants. None of these seem to work in any predictable manner. A drug used to treat hypertension called Clonidine, has shown some success in preventing bruxism, but comes with a worrisome side effect—a fall in blood pressure.

Occasionally, painkillers and anti-inflammatory drugs are needed to treat pain in the temporomandibular joint, or even toothache, caused by severe episodes of tooth grinding. Warm compresses over the joint also help at such times.

Psychological Measures

The only tangible cause of bruxism that can be addressed effectively is psychological stress. Its alleviation will require conscious effort on your part, as there are many ways out.

The first step is to be aware of, and to acknowledge the presence of tension. Stress is usually the cumulative product of a compounding of petty irritants, anger, resentment and frustrations that occur through our daily lives. These need to be dissipated before they grow to dangerous proportions.

Relaxation techniques like yoga, meditation, hobbies, exercise, holidays, bonding with family and friends—all of these help us to let off steam. Lifestyle changes may need to be incorporated to accomplish some of these measures. When negative emotions are not allowed to mount, the tendency to brux the teeth reduces automatically.

Some people may need the help of psychological counselors to put them on the right track for managing their stress.

Bruxism is a complex condition, which causes disturbance to sleep, generates muscular pain, and much damage to the teeth and jaws. Your dentist can help diagnose this problem, and relieve many of its symptoms. However, the permanent solution may lie in the way you handle your thoughts and emotions. Relax, sit back and enjoy life: don't let bruxism become a millstone around your neck!

Chapter 12

Fillings:
Restore and Rejoice

A modern-day scenario: you rush out from work to make it in time for your dental appointment to have that aching tooth filled. Take heart, people have been doing this for millennia! Archaeologists have found drilled teeth in remains dating back to 7000 BC (from the Indus Valley civilization). They believe that bow-driven tools were used to drill holes in teeth—not for filling them—but to drive evil spirits away!

Modern day dentistry, thankfully, employs state-of-the-art technology, equipment and skillful professionals to treat dental decay!

Cavity Treatment Across Time: Down Memory Lane

Cavities in teeth have been around for thousands of years, with numerous materials serving as fillings. Beeswax seems to be one of the oldest options ever used, nearly 6,500 years ago, possibly in an attempt to make a cracked tooth less sensitive. Other substances included stone chips, cork, plant resins or gums and various metals.

Metallic fillings have been around for ages. Gold being one of the early favourites, it became a status symbol, with people literally putting their money where their mouth was!

In the last couple of centuries, silver has been the material of choice. Silver paste, as a tooth filling, was known in China more than 2,000 years ago; but the modern silver amalgam was first formulated by a Parisian, Auguste Taveau, in 1816, using silver coins and mercury.

The original formula underwent several modifications, till the grand ol' daddy of dentistry, Dr G.V. Black, perfected the proportions of silver, tin and mercury in the mix. Silver amalgam is still used today, although its virtues are shadowed by controversy.

The quest for a 'white' filling led to the development of silicate cement in the late nineteenth century, the forerunner of many of the 'cosmetic' filling formulas available today.

Signs of Cavity Formation: The Hole Story

So how would you know whether you need a filling? A filling reconstructs that portion of the tooth, which has gone to rot or has broken away in an injury. Small cavities may not trigger any symptoms, as the outermost layer of our teeth is insensitive, owing to which many sufferers tend to ignore it. But, if you visit the dentist at this stage, the treatment will be conservative, and a small filling can often do the trick.

Very often, cavities form between two teeth, leading to the jamming of food particles in this space.

As the cavity dredges deeper, you may experience sensitivity to cold and hot foods and beverages, as well as to sweets. If the decay is not too extensive, and hasn't yet damaged the inner pulp, this sensation will normally last just a few seconds. The reaction, though not debilitating, is troublesome, and is often described as a 'shock-like' twinge.

In deeper cavities, the temporary tenderness can soon

turn into persistent ache when it approaches the delicate pulp within the tooth. At this stage, a filling might still be possible, with an extra protective layer (a liner) to soothe the pulp, before applying the permanent filling.

Ignoring the cavity and pain at this point allows the damage to progress, and you would need to turn to Chapter Thirteen to know more about the option of a root canal treatment!

At the Dentist's: Step-by-Step

Once you do visit your dentist with a cavity, there are a few standard steps that will be followed.

Scan and Probe

The first step in the filling process begins with the dentist taking a close look at the teeth. Using a small mouth mirror and a sharp, pointed instrument known as an explorer, the dentist checks each tooth to identify decay. An air or water spray may be used to flush the surfaces clean to aid this examination. Occasionally, a safe staining dye is used to highlight the rotted areas.

X-rays are also routinely employed to diagnose the presence of cavities, especially on hidden surfaces of the teeth. For doubtful areas, the dentist may use a powerful lamp, which can show up decayed areas of the tooth as dark shadows (this is called trans-illumination). These days, laser-based probes are available to scan the teeth for early stages of spoilage, which are otherwise undetectable.

Drilling

Once the decayed tooth is identified, it is first numbed with the help of local anaesthesia. The filling procedure is initiated only after complete and profound numbness is established, in order to prevent discomfort during the process.

The dentist then removes the rot, which is usually softened due to the germ warfare—you may know this operation by the name of drilling (the dentist's term for this is 'cavity preparation').

Dental drills have come a long way from the centuries old hand-powered versions! Over time, more refined instruments made their appearance—some driven through clockwork mechanisms, others by coil springs. In 1790, George Washington's dentist, John Greenwood, modified his mother's spinning wheel and foot treadle to run a drill, inventing the world's first dental foot engine! After many incarnations and reincarnations, modern-day drills have evolved into their high-speed precision avatars.

Today's dental clinic is equipped with the standard pneumatic drills, known as 'airotors', which can function at speeds of up to 4,00,000 revolutions per minute. The drill bits, which fit onto the air rotor, are small diamond-coated points, or made of tough tungsten carbide, both of which can pierce the hard tooth substance in minutes. The running of the pneumatic drill generates heat, so water is sprayed through it to act as a coolant—ejected from the mouth via a sterile tip connected to a suction machine.

Generally, people are terrified of the high-pitched whine of the drill, associating it with pain. However, most cavities today are treated under the effect of local anaesthesia, which makes the exercise painless. Modern airotor drills have also been redesigned to work efficiently with low sound levels.

The drilling process is meant to remove the decayed portions of the tooth. Occasionally, people feel that the very tiny cavity they came with became massive after the dentist drilled into it! This is because most of us cannot imagine the extent of the decay, or the depth of the cavity. Often what you see as a black spot can, in reality, be just the tip of the iceberg, with a large decayed area existing under the surface.

Earlier, dentists strictly followed Dr G.V. Black's original guidelines for drilling. This necessitated a definitive shape and depth to the cavity preparation for receiving the filling. It meant that dentists would even remove sound, healthy parts of the tooth, as they wanted to avoid future decay along its natural grooves!

With the evolution of newer materials and techniques, the practices have changed—today the focus is on removal of the decayed areas only. The emphasis is on being minimally invasive—in other words, to preserve as much of the natural tooth as possible. Dentists also advise and encourage good oral hygiene, and periodic monitoring of the fillings to prevent recurrence of decay.

Newer innovations include air-abrasion machines, and even lasers are used to remove tooth decay.

Flushing Out the Rot

Once the rot is out and the cavity prepared, the debris is flushed away. Generally, dentists also apply a disinfectant to the prepared surfaces to eliminate any bacterial infection. After this, the tooth is rinsed and dried with an air spray, and kept isolated, or free from contact with the tongue, lips or cheek, as it is necessary to prevent the saliva from wetting and contaminating the tooth. This can be achieved in a few ways:

- By simply placing rolls of cotton around the tooth
- By holding a rubber dam, which is a sheet of rubber,

around the tooth with special clamps. (These are used extensively in the West, not only for isolation, but also to prevent anything from going down the throat. In India, its use is rather infrequent.)
* By moving away the lip, tongue and cheek with plastic devices called retractors, combined with high-powered suctioning to keep off moisture

Often, decay leaves a large deficit in the tooth, eating away one or more of the cavity walls. This could allow the filling to overflow the confines of the cavity, leading to future problems such as damage to the gums. To prevent this, dentists deploy a temporary retaining barrier called a matrix, to ensure that the filling remains within the natural contours of the tooth.

Time to Fill Up

A wide range of filling materials is now available to treat different types of cavities, and the various situations in which they occur.

Here is what you ought to expect from a filling:

* It should be strong enough to handle the load of biting and chewing.
* It needs to blend in with the colour of your own teeth, especially if in a visible area such as a front tooth.
* It needs to be durable and long lasting.
* It should be safe enough to be placed in the mouth, without harming the tooth, gums and the delicate oral tissues.
* Its application should be fast and comfortable.
* It needs to set quickly into place, allowing you to use the tooth soon.
* It should be affordable!

Before applying the filling, a protective layer known as a base or liner is placed in the deepest recesses of the prepared cavity. This guards the delicate pulp within from thermal (hot/cold) sensations, and insulates it from any potential irritation by the filling itself.

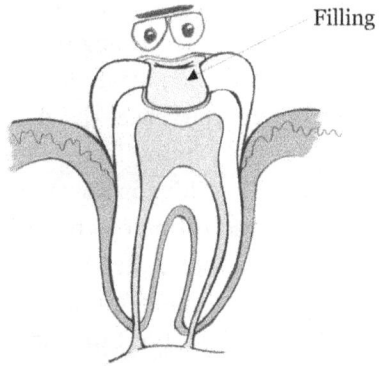

Filling

The choice of filling is determined by two considerations: your preference with respect to the colour (tooth-coloured or metallic), and its cost; and the dentist's judgment of the type that will best suit you.

Gold

Till date, gold is considered one of the best fillings, as it is the most compatible with the body. Compressed gold foil can be filled directly into the cavity in several layers. It is extremely durable, wearing away only at the same rate as your tooth. However, its prohibitive cost makes it unpopular, creating the need for a more cost-effective option.

Silver

For close to 200 years, silver has been the most popular filling material in the form of a silver amalgam—a powdered alloy of silver, tin, zinc and copper with mercury. The mixing is done just prior to the procedure, to keep it pliable, similar in consistency to stiff putty. It was traditionally compounded in a mortar and pestle, but now small machines named amalgamators execute the proportioning and blending. Some dentists prefer a pre-proportioned alloy-and-mercury capsule, which is mixed in a dedicated device just before use.

After protecting the cavity with a cement liner, the filling is compacted inside it and sculpted to the shape of the tooth. Before you leave, the dentist will check that the filling is at the right biting level.

The filling hardens over the next few hours, and it is best to avoid eating on this tooth for at least twelve hours. In the next session, the dentist will polish the filling to achieve a glossy, shining surface. This mended tooth is now ready to perform all the functions of the original one.

Here are the advantages of this popular filling:

- It is inexpensive.
- It is durable, easily lasting fifteen to twenty years and more.
- It is most forgiving of the variables in which different dentists use it—in other words, it is less technique-sensitive.
- It has good strength, enough to withstand the chewing forces of the back teeth.
- It works well even when there is slight contamination during the procedure due to moisture or saliva.

All that said, silver fillings have yet been losing their sheen over the last few decades, with the availability of newer alternatives. Some of its disadvantages have contributed to this. For one, many of us don't like the metallic look of silver—and obviously, it is not usable in the front teeth. Besides, a greater amount of drilling is required to create the requisite space for the filling, as the material is not strong enough in thin layers. This means that more healthy portions of the tooth need to be drilled out. Not surprisingly, two sittings are required for the completion of the procedure, as the filling cannot be polished immediately.

There are other disadvantages, too. The material does not bond with the tooth—this can cause leakage between them. Silver fillings undergo corrosion, and it is these accumulated by-products that eventually seal the leaky margins. Over time, these fillings can cause a blackish discolouration of the healthy portions of the tooth.

Significantly, being less biocompatible than gold, silver fillings may cause irritation or allergic responses when in contact with the delicate gums and oral tissues.

The most controversial aspect of such fillings, however, is the use of mercury in the amalgam! Health concerns about mercury came sharply into focus in the early part of the twentieth century. The German scientist, Alfred Stock, conducted several studies and concluded that certain health problems were related to the mercury vapours being released from dental fillings. He had his own silver fillings removed, and advised his friends to do so too. His findings, coupled with this radical step, forced the hand of many health agencies, which began doubting the wondrous qualities of silver amalgam fillings.

Mercury was labelled as a toxin, causing serious health issues—called heavy-metal poisoning—when ingested. Dentists were asked not to use these fillings in children, pregnant women and patients with kidney ailments. The doubts also resulted in banning it in many Scandinavian countries, and in some states within the USA as well.

While there has been no conclusive evidence of its harmfulness when used in silver amalgam, the controversy rages on. Despite this, silver amalgam continues to be popular as a filling for molars and premolars.

Light-cured Composite Resin (LCCR)

In the olden days, tooth-coloured fillings weren't around, and people would flaunt gold fillings even on their front teeth! However, the need for a more camouflaged filling, especially for the front teeth, was always felt.

The first of the tooth-coloured fillings—the silicate cements—made its appearance around the end of the nineteenth century. Silicate glass powders and phosphoric acid were mixed together, and the resulting paste filled into the prepared tooth cavity, where it would set into a hard, white filling. This substance, however, was pretty harsh on the delicate pulp, and gradually fell into disuse.

Years of research and refinement have finally yielded today's tooth-coloured, 'cosmetic' filling, known as the light-cured composite resin (LCCR). Apart from being visually pleasing, this material has a critical quality: it is strong enough to withstand the chewing forces even in thin layers. This means that dentists can be highly conservative with the drilling, restricting it to the bare minimum. Thus it also lives up to today's requirement for saving the healthy areas of the tooth.

There are three major advantages in using LCCR. For one, it contains hard filler particles embedded in an acrylic resin base. In the form of a thick paste, it is available in a variety of shades, which can match any natural tooth colour.

Secondly, the presence of certain chemicals in the material, called 'photoinitiators', causes it to harden when exposed to light, in just twenty seconds. (To activate this reaction, dentists use a hand-held light-cure machine, which is essentially a device with a powerful halogen lamp or LED light source. Special filters allow only the blue part of normal light to come through a fine tip attached to it known as a light probe.)

Lastly, LCCR needs to be bonded onto the tooth, and this is achieved by using a thin, glue-like material known as a bonding agent. Older versions of this agent required prior treatment of the cavity surface with an acid to roughen it. Since the latest bonding agents incorporate an acid, that step is avoided.

Accordingly, this is how the filling process goes. After the cavity is prepared, the tooth is isolated and a suitable liner applied inside to protect the tooth. The glue-like bonding agent is then applied, and hardened by exposure to the glare of the light-cure machine.

Next, the dentist selects the shade of resin most closely matching the colour of the tooth being treated. The first layer of this material is then placed in the cavity, and set into place or 'cured', by exposure to the blue light. The cavity is slowly filled up, in similar fashion, layer-by-layer. Once the filling is duly completed, the material is hard enough to be trimmed and polished, to mesh with the contours of the tooth.

Lastly, a final sealer (similar to a glossy varnish) is applied on the filling to prevent the likelihood of staining and leakages.

So here's the good side of a LCCR filling:

- Being tooth-coloured, it creates lifelike fillings, perfectly blending in with the tooth.
- This material enables the dentist to be highly conservative with the drilling, resulting in better preservation of the healthy parts of the tooth.
- Since it is bonded to the tooth, it doesn't suffer from leakage at the joints.
- It is time-saving, as the filling process can be completed and polished in a single sitting.

- It is free of mercury, and therefore totally innocent of its potential hazards.
- Being strong even in thin layers, it can also be used to repair minor chips and breaks in teeth.
- Composite fillings are repairable; it is possible to add to an existing filling, without having to remove it.

There's always a flip side, so here are the concerns regarding LCCR fillings. For one, they are not as strong as silver amalgam, especially if the filling area is large, and are expensive—much more than the cost of silver fillings. Worse, the fillings tend to stain, especially if they are not polished well.

Also, the outcome is extremely technique sensitive, and relies a lot on the dentist's skill and experience, and the manner in which the filling is placed.

The chances of recurring decay along the filling are increased, as some composite resins shrink when they harden. The resin can also irritate the delicate pulp inside the tooth, especially in the case of deeper cavities. Indeed, there are concerns about the potential toxicity of the acrylic resins in the material.

If time is of the essence, you need to know that compared to silver amalgam, it takes more time to complete an LCCR filling procedure—this results in a longer sitting for you!

Glass Ionomer

This is also a tooth-coloured filling, comprising a glass powder mixed with polyacrylic acid. Let's list the advantages:

- It has a unique property—it bonds chemically to the tooth surface, without the need of any additional bonding agent!
- Conventional versions of this material harden

chemically when mixed, and don't need any light-curing.

- It also releases fluoride, protecting the filled tooth from recurrent decay.
- Glass ionomer fillings can be completed quickly too, and are less expensive than LCCR fillings.

On the other hand, it is not as strong as composite resin, and cannot be placed in the load-bearing teeth. While it is white, it is not very attractive as it tends to look opaque, and doesn't carry a good surface polish.

Having said that, there are some specific areas where it works well:

- For fillings in milk teeth, where the demands for strength and aesthetics are lower (its fluoride-releasing quality is also deeply desirable in children's teeth)
- For filling cavities along root surfaces exposed by gum recession, especially in geriatric patients
- Occasionally, as a base under the LCCR filling to protect the precious pulp from irritation caused by composite resin

In an attempt to increase the strength of the glass ionomer powder, a material known as 'cermet' was developed, which incorporated the silver-filling alloy into it. However, it still suffered from being weaker than silver amalgam, and with its unattractiveness due to the dark colour, it has since become obsolete.

Newer versions of glass ionomer have tried to incorporate some of the advantages of LCCR, and are termed as resin-modified glass ionomer cements. They are stronger, and have a better surface-finish, while retaining the quality of fluoride-release. Besides the times when glass-ionomer is conventionally used, resin-modified glass ionomer cements can qualify for minor fillings in the permanent front teeth.

Prefabricated Fillings

In some instances, after the rot is drilled away, the remaining tooth structure is inadequate to support a normal filling. In this case, the dentist takes an impression of the teeth to make a mould of the prepared tooth, and sends it to a dental laboratory with relevant instructions.

The laboratory technicians then make a customized filling using gold or porcelain—the inlay or onlay—which will fit precisely inside or onto the prepared tooth. This is then stuck to the tooth with adhesive dental cement.

An inlay is recommended by your dentist if the decay has devoured a large part of the chewing surface of your tooth, but left most of the outer walls still intact.

Or, your dentist may recommend an onlay if the decay has damaged the cusps of the back teeth. This replicates exactly the shape of the natural cusps.

Inlays and onlays have far more strength than normal fillings, and their shape can be precisely contoured in the laboratory. However, the cost factor increases, due to escalated procedures and laboratory costs.

Home Care for the Filled Cavity: Don't Shut and Forget

Fillings are hugely successful in restoring teeth that have suffered damage due to tooth decay. Irrespective of the type of filling, it is imperative that it is monitored and checked every six months. A filled tooth *can* develop further decay along the filled surface or on a new surface. A filling treats existing decay; it *does not* guarantee freedom from future decay!

A tooth filling is like a repair job. And like all repair jobs, it needs extra care and maintenance from your side. Every filled tooth needs the same oral hygiene care as your other healthy, natural teeth. If you stick to the programme of brushing, flossing and bi-annual dental checks, you can ensure the continued good health of not only your filled teeth, but of all the other teeth as well. If a filled tooth is cared for, it is less likely to require frequent replacement or advanced treatment for years.

In conclusion, there is a wide range of options when it comes to filling teeth that are damaged by decay. Function, aesthetics and cost are the main factors that influence the choice of filling. Modern materials ensure that fillings can be done quickly and painlessly. They restore form and function to damaged teeth, and can serve well for years with good follow-up care.

Chapter 13

Root Canal Treatment: Navigating Down Under

As far back into the past as 200 BC, ancient physicians understood the importance of saving a Nabatean warrior's incisor tooth. In Israel's Negev desert, archaeologists have found radiological evidence of a metal wire that had been implanted inside the tooth, within the thin canal running through the root. It is the first evidence of a root canal treatment! Since such expertise was not locally available in ancient times, it is assumed that Roman doctors would have performed this advanced treatment.

The Evolution of Root Canal Treatment: Of Worms and Other Horrors

As we know, as far back as 5,000 years ago, the Sumerians attributed tooth decay to 'worms' attacking the teeth. This belief persisted over the ages in different forms, but it was only late in the eighteenth century that Pierre Fauchard, considered the father of modern dentistry, dispelled the worm theory. With the help of a microscope he proved that there were indeed no worms in decayed teeth. He also described, for the first time, the delicate tissues within the tooth—the dental pulp— and suggested its removal to treat severe toothaches.

However, until recent times, when fillings couldn't provide relief, the next line of treatment for the ill-fated tooth was extraction. Over the last couple of centuries, many attempts were made to preserve teeth by cleaning up the damaged pulp in various ways. This ranged from using hot instruments to cauterize the tissue, to applying different chemicals like arsenic, formalin and phenol to deaden it.

These procedures were largely associated with excruciating pain, due to inadequate or no application of local anaesthesia. This is the basis for many horror stories accompanying the treatment of dental pulp!

Today, it can be safely considered passé to talk about one's frightful stories of root canal treatment, because it has become widely known that this *doesn't* instigate pain—and that it actually *eliminates* pain! In fact, it has proved itself to be an extremely successful line of treatment, as the tooth is saved from being extracted, and continues to function just like other normal teeth.

Understanding Root Canal Treatment: Deep Inside the Tooth

Root canal treatment is currently an exceedingly common procedure, but most people have only a vague notion about how it goes. Therefore, one of the regular questions asked at every dental clinic is, 'What exactly is root canal treatment?'

If you refresh your memory about the structure of the tooth, you will remember that lying at its very core is a soft, delicate tissue known as 'dental pulp'. This essentially contains the blood and nerve supplies, and is completely surrounded by the hard layers of the tooth. The pulp has a larger, bulb-like section protected within the crown. It also has a thin hair-like passage in the root area, which courses through a narrow, tubular space called the *root canal*. This is what has lent its name to the procedure known as root canal treatment.

The correct technical name for root canal treatment is endodontic treatment—treatment of tissues that lie *inside* the tooth. When the dental pulp suffers irreversible damage, the only way to save the tooth is to totally remove those tissues, and to refill the empty space with a suitable substitute. This is the simplest description of endodontic or root canal treatment.

There are many ways in which dental pulp can encounter extreme damage. The commonest reason for serious harm is a glaring cavity. When cavities are not treated in the early stages, they travel far inside the tooth, till they reach the pulp. Such deep-seated decay can also emerge beneath existing fillings or crowns. Bacteria in such situations induce damage and devastation to the pulp.

Teeth afflicted by trauma or breakage due to a blow or other accidents, can also suffer injury to the pulp. Moreover, some teeth develop deep cracks due to habits like paan-chewing, or tooth grinding. If these cracks reach the pulp, it becomes vulnerable to hurt.

Severe gum disease can allow bacterial infection to reach and affect the pulp through the tip or side of the root.

In addition, if a tooth needs to be prepared for a crown or a bridge procedure, this can eventually result in hurting the pulp. Such teeth may need to be pre-emptively treated by root canal treatment.

Occasionally, the entire pulp tissue dies out, leading to a collection of pus or an abscess at the tip of the root.

Signs You Might Need Root Canal Treatment: Oh, That Feeling!

Teeth in which the pulp has been severely damaged can be excessively painful! Here are some of the typical symptoms of distress:

- Excruciating, sharp, shooting pain in the tooth, lasting more than a few minutes without any hot or cold or food triggers
- Toothache that worsens at night—one of the classical symptoms that sufferers complain about (the throbbing pain is due to an increase in pressure within an infected tooth when in a prone position. Of course, if one were to take an afternoon siesta, the same throbbing pain would attack then too.)
- Repeated episodes of lingering pain upon eating hot and cold food items
- A constant dull, throbbing toothache after eating
- Intolerable pain, mitigated only buy holding ice-water in the mouth, in direct contact with the affected tooth (such pain could be on account of damage to the pulp that leads to an abscess at the tip of the root.)
- Lingering infections at the tips of the roots, which spread slowly within the jawbone (if the pulp has totally died out, one could be troubled with chronic infections; these could seek to find an opening into the mouth through the bone, leading to a boil on the gum.)
- Painful swellings on the face or inside the mouth

Very often, one tends to postpone seeing the dentist, dreading the stories of pain connected with root canal treatment. Self-medication with pain killers is common, but it only offers a temporary reprieve.

Routine dental checks can help detect problems before they turn painful. In any case, it is always best to see the dentist as soon as symptoms of toothache manifest, rather than allowing matters to worsen. Once the dentist completes the clinical examination, you may be prescribed the correct pain relieving medication and even a course of antibiotics, if necessary.

For hyper-anxious people, anti-stress premedication may be prescribed prior to the procedure to allay apprehensions. The best pain control is actually achieved by the root canal treatment procedure itself—in fact, a number of people don't even require painkillers after this treatment, and the toothache vanishes!

The Procedure for Root Canal Treatment: Filing It Away

Root canal treatment is a well-structured procedure, involving a series of steps.

Anaesthesia

The key to achieving a painless root canal treatment is this— the tooth is first numbed with a local anaesthetic. Occasionally, when there is pus collection in and around the tooth, the effectiveness of anaesthesia is reduced, and one is likely to experience pain during the treatment. In such cases, your dentist will first counter the infection with pre-medications, like antibiotics and analgesics for a painfree procedure. As a rule, the root canal procedure is initiated only after complete numbness in the tooth is established. (Some totally dead teeth may need no anaesthesia, but your dentist is the best judge of this.)

X-rays

An X-ray of the tooth is taken before starting the root canal treatment procedure. This helps the dentist understand the structure of the tooth, and to assess the length of the roots. X-rays will also show up any abnormality that might exist in the roots and the surrounding areas, as well as the presence of infections at the root tips.

Isolation

The tooth to be treated is isolated, preferably with a rubber dam, as described in Chapter Twelve, to shield the mouth tissues against chemicals used during the root canal treatment procedure. It keeps the treatment zone free of bacterial contamination, and also prevents the chances of any of the small instruments employed from being inadvertently inhaled or swallowed.

Preparation

Regular dental drills are first deployed to remove all the decomposed portions of the tooth, and then to gain access into the hollows within, which contain the dental pulp.

Next, a thin, needle-like instrument known as a *hand file*, detects and enters the fine, hair-like root canals. Some teeth have a single canal (such as the upper incisors), others have two (like the upper first premolars), and a few have three or more (as in the molars).

Specialized drill bits called rotary files, which run on high-powered low speed drills, then clean out the damaged contents within the roots. The canals are also gradually enlarged with progressively larger drills.

Some dentists prefer hand files for the entire process,

Root Canal Treatment

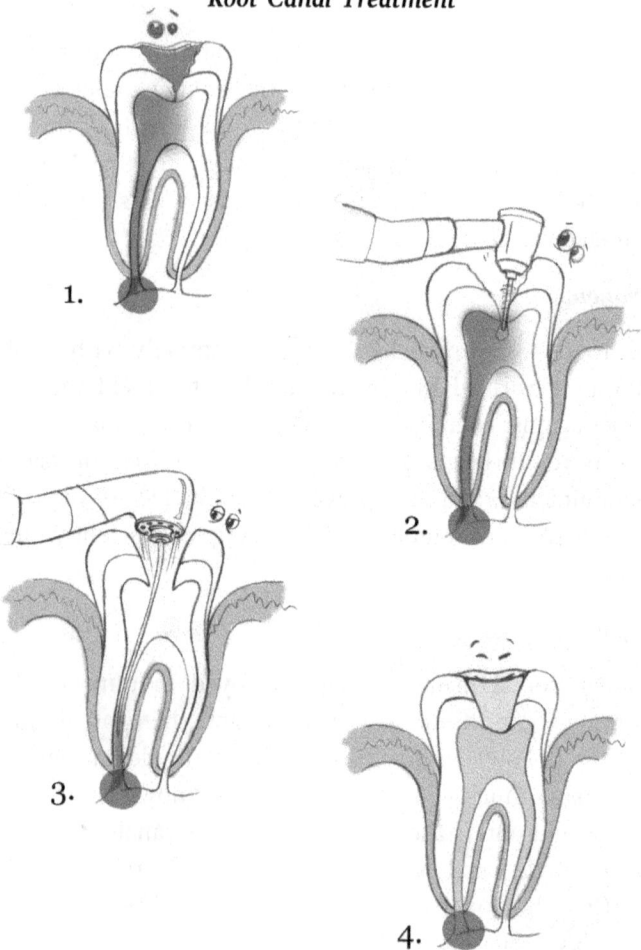

but most have switched to the rotary file systems. Hand files are still practical in some situations—such as when navigating through curved roots.

The dentist may use magnifying eyewear known as loupes, or even an endodontic microscope for better views of the minute root canal openings. Throughout the process, dentists use chemical gels known as lubricants, to facilitate this cleaning and shaping process.

The debris generated by the drilling is also dissolved and flushed out with chemical solutions such as sodium hypochlorite.

The roots need to be cleaned meticulously till their tips, for which dentists rely on modern equipment called apex locators, to establish and confirm the length of the root canals. An X-ray is taken to confirm that the root is perfectly cleaned till the end, only then is it finally ready to receive the filling.

Currently, most dentists proceed to complete the final stage of filling in the same session, popularly known as a single-sitting RCT. On the rare occasion that the dentist may postpone the final filling for a subsequent sitting, he places an antibacterial substance within the roots, covering it with a temporary filling for the interim.

Filling

The process of filling the cleaned and shaped canals is called obturation. The metal wire found in the warrior from 200 BC would be known as an obturation material. In fact, silver wires (called silver cones) have been trusted until recent times for this function.

Gutta-percha, a rubber-like material, is now the preferred choice of dentists the world over. The solidified latex from the sap of a South American tree, it is an inert material, highly biocompatible with human tissues and suitably modified for use. Flexible, or softened by heat application if need be, it is manufactured in a conical shape, almost corresponding to that of the root canal. Called a gutta-percha point, it is available in varying lengths and thicknesses to adapt to canals with differing dimensions.

Once the canal is ready for the filling, it is dried with thin 'paper points' which also follow the shape of the canal.

To avoid any gaps between the gutta-percha point and the walls of the canals, a sealer in the form of a thin paste is first introduced into the canals. (This paste hardens up in a few hours.)

Then, a main gutta-percha point (known as a master cone) is placed inside the prepared root canal, going right down till the root tip.

Additional smaller points may then be positioned alongside, for which space is created by a packing instrument known as a spreader. Multiple points may be needed in a canal to ensure a tightly packed fit.

The projecting ends of the points at the crown front are finally trimmed, softened with a heated instrument and smoothed down.

Newer techniques include the heat-softened (thermoplastic) gutta-percha, which is inserted in the canal under pressure with a dedicated dispensing gun and needle. Recently, a few resin-based systems have also made their appearance, eliminating the need for gutta percha.

This process effectively seals off the canal at the root tip. A good seal is also needed at the crown end of the filling, which is usually done with a glass ionomer base. Once the root canal is fully secured in this manner, the tooth is ready for its final restoration—the filling in the decayed (now empty) portions of the tooth.

As it may remain tender for a few days, the dentist will usually reduce the length of the treated tooth so that it doesn't come in contact with the opposing one when chewing. Since it would also continue to be numb, it is not advisable to eat from that side for a few hours till the sensation returns. An analgesic can be taken to avoid any post-treatment pain, and continued for a few days as necessary.

As a matter of fact, most folks who undergo root canal treatment soon go off painkillers. As mentioned earlier, root canal treatment doesn't activate pain, it eliminates pain!

Fixing the Crown

After root canal treatment, the tooth loses its internal blood supply, which was cardinal in keeping it moist and hydrated from within. The moistness had conferred a degree of resilience to the hard tooth structure, thereby allowing it to withstand the heavy forces of chewing.

Thus, dentists advise that any chewing tooth having undergone root canal treatment needs to be protected with a crown, because the lack of moisture desiccates it, making it liable to fractures. So, while the tooth might look strong, it becomes brittle and can crack under the pressure of chewing.

A crown or cap, is a dental restoration that completely covers the visible portion of a tooth (or an implant). Composed of strong material, which is resistant to breakage, it can keep the tooth functioning for years.

To accommodate a crown, the dentist first whittles down the tooth from all sides by a high-speed dental drill or airotor. A prescribed shape is accomplished which also provides an accurate margin, or step, on which the edges of the crown will sit.

After preparing the tooth thus, the dentist takes an impression of the teeth, with a paste-like material held against them till it sets. A substance similar to plaster-of-paris is then employed to replicate a model or cast from this impression. This is then sent to a specialized dental laboratory, which fabricates the crown.

Crowns can be made entirely of metal, such as a nickel-chromium alloy, or even with alloys of precious metals like gold, palladium, etc. Tooth-coloured crowns are formed by covering an inner metal core with a coating of porcelain (ceramic) or of resin. Recent developments include metal-free crowns, in which a zirconia core replaces the metallic one. Zirconia is a white, non-metallic, rugged material displaying remarkably high strength. Crowns made entirely of zirconia, are also now available.

The dentist receives the prescribed crown from the dental laboratory, checks the fit, shape, and colour, and verifies its contact points with neighbouring and opposing teeth. It is then permanently fixed into place with strong dental cements—and the tooth is now ready to get back to work!

The Success and Failure Rates of Root Canal Treatments: The Highs and Lows

A question often asked by patients at a dental clinic is, 'What's the life of my tooth after a root canal treatment?' Over the years, root canal treatment has proven itself to be an eminently successful form of treatment. In fact, studies have placed the success rate between 86 to 97 per cent! With the right precautions, routine maintenance, and regular checkups, a tooth with root canal treatment can last a lifetime.

However, there *are* instances where the treatment does not fully succeed, or fails to prevent pain and infection. Some of these are:

- When the cleaning and preparation of the roots is not performed thoroughly enough, leaving behind dead or

infected tissue
- If the tooth has curved roots or blocked canals within, not allowing thorough cleaning
- If the final root filling or obturation falls short of the root tip
- If one or more canals remained untreated as their openings could not be found
- If the tooth has extra 'lateral canals' branching off from the main canals, which could not be cleaned and filled
- If any of the root canal treatment instruments, especially files, break inside the thin canals and cannot be retrieved
- When recurrent caries occurs under a filling or a crown, compromising the seal of the root canal filling
- When severe gum disease allows infection to enter the root canals
- If the tooth has an unusual anatomy, such as additional roots or canals which could not be discovered
- If the final filling was postponed, resulting in re-infection within the root canals.
- If the root fractures due to the chewing load

Many of these failures can be addressed by re-treating the tooth, and by correcting the cause of the failure. This is usually more complex than the original root canal treatment, but if performed successfully, it can ensure good long-term success.

Some of these failed cases may require surgical procedures known as endodontic surgery, to eliminate the infection. This often involves removal of the tip of the infected root, and placing a filling inside the cut portion to seal it. Some dentists perform these operations themselves, while others may recommend the services of a specialist (known as an endodontist), to treat such complicated cases.

Rarely, a tooth with a failed root canal treatment may not be amenable to re-treatment or surgical correction, and will need to be extracted and replaced with an artificial tooth.

Root Canal Treatment for Kids: Child's Play?

Children, too, could need endodontic treatment!

As we know, milk teeth are crucial, and need to be preserved till their designated time of shedding. If they contract deep decay, leading to damage of the dental pulp, they become candidates for endodontic treatment.

If the dentist finds the pulp in the roots still healthy, and only that of the crown portion damaged, a procedure known as a pulpotomy (akin to a half root canal treatment, as mentioned earlier) may be implemented. Here, the damaged pulp is removed and a filling is inserted, to restore the tooth.

If the damage to the pulp extends into the root portions as well, and if the tooth is a long way from its destined time of exfoliation, a proper root canal treatment is necessitated. Often, parents avoid this treatment for a milk tooth, arguing that it will fall off anyway and be replaced by a permanent tooth. Yet, if root canal treatment *is* executed on a damaged milk tooth, it can help the child in chewing better, and thereby help in her overall growth and wellbeing.

In milk teeth, the cleaning of the roots is done in a similar fashion as for permanent teeth. However, for the final root filling or obturation, resorbable materials are substituted for gutta-percha, as they need to melt away along with the root of the milk tooth during the shedding process.

Most milk molars need to be restored with crowns after root canal treatment, and stainless steel crowns are the recommended option. They fall off with the tooth, and will not need to be removed before that.

Permanent teeth in children may also require root canal treatment, either due to deep decay or an injury that damages the pulp. The treatment procedure is carried out in the standard manner as described earlier.

In some instances, when root canal treatment is necessary for permanent front teeth—usually the incisors, having sustained an injury, typically from contact sports—and if the root tip (apex) is not formed or fully closed, the root canal treatment is done in two stages.

The first artificially facilitates the closure of the root tip, in a process called apexification, by inserting a calcium hydroxide paste into the cleaned canal. In the second stage, after a few months or even a year, the root canal is revisited, the canals cleaned and shaped, and the routine root canal treatment is completed.

Root canal treatment is truly a boon for saving teeth, which would otherwise be consigned to the extraction forceps. It is a time-tested, predictable and extremely successful mode of treatment. The icing on the cake is that, with all the refinements that this procedure has undergone over time, it is painless too!

Chapter 14

Dental Extractions:
Pluck-me-not

One of the foremost reasons for dreading the dentist can be attributed to our history! A Mesopotamian text from 1800 BC, the Code of Hammurabi, mentions tooth extractions as an efficient means for punishment! Obviously, it would be a form of torture, as it was not until the mid-nineteenth century that anaesthesia was introduced for the removal of teeth!

The patroness of dentistry, Saint Appolonia, was subjected to the forcible extraction of all her teeth before being burnt alive in the third century BC. Many who were suffering toothache and had to undergo painful extractions, were told to pray to her and think of her miserable death!

In the early days, it was barbers who practiced dentistry, and who didn't mind using surgical instruments for tooth extractions. Of course, these were simple gadgets like Guy de Chauliac's lever-based tool called the dental pelican (as it resembled a bird's beak).

As can be understood, these

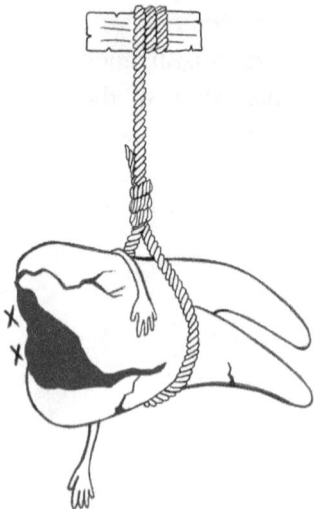

were mostly trauma-inducing instruments, which wrenched the tooth out of the jaw. Apart from their gross inefficiency in doing this job, they managed to damage the gums and the surrounding areas too. This method was practiced from the fourteenth to the eighteenth centuries, till replaced by Alexander Monro's 'tooth key'. Late in the nineteenth century, the dental forceps were invented, modern adaptations of which are still current.

Yet, here we are in the twenty-first century, still fearing to visit the modern dental clinic for tooth extractions, done under local anaesthesia, in peaceful and hygienic clinics, with sterilized instruments and performed by skilled and qualified professionals! In these times, the fear of extraction is an unreasonable one, but its origins are surely deep-seated enough from the nightmares of the past.

When Teeth Need Extraction: The Case for the Prosecution

Today, with so many advanced treatment options, why would we still need teeth to be pulled out? Sadly, many of them suffer damage that is beyond the capacity of even the best dental procedures to restore, and so mandate removal. Here are the major examples:

- A tooth that is so badly decayed and broken down that it cannot be repaired
- Teeth that are extremely loose, due to the last stages of gum disease
- Teeth that are hopelessly fractured, such as below the gum level or in the case of a vertical splitting of the root
- Teeth with very widespread infections, which even endodontic treatment can't eliminate

- Teeth with failed root canal treatment or endodontic treatment, where re-treatment is not viable
- During treatment for cancer in the head, face or neck, when some infected teeth need to be removed prior to radiation, to prevent complications in the jawbones
- For budgetary reasons—to save on the costs of fillings or endodontic treatment (this is usually against the doctor's advice, and is an unwise decision)

Occasionally, healthy teeth are removed to facilitate other treatment procedures, such as:

- Orthodontic treatment, to create space for realigning the remaining teeth
- Teeth that exist in the line of a jaw fracture, which may impede the healing process
- Teeth that may be severely inclined, or otherwise obstructing the plan for replacing lost teeth with dentures
- Teeth that may look ungainly due to their angulation or position, removal of which can facilitate cosmetic treatment processes
- Extra teeth (called supernumerary teeth), which may be detrimental to maintaining the health of the remaining teeth

Some teeth need to be removed surgically, due to stalled eruptions:

- Wisdom teeth, whose eruption is blocked or incomplete due to improper angulation inside the jaw (these are called 'impacted wisdom teeth', which often lead to infections, or even decay in the neighbouring teeth)
- Permanent canines, which are stuck within the jaw due

to adverse angulation
* Extra or supernumerary teeth, which may prevent the eruption of other normal teeth

Anaesthesia and Tooth Extraction: There's Safety in Numbing

All of us would like the procedure to be a painless one! This is easily achieved by numbing the tooth with anaesthesia. In India, dentists are legally prohibited from administering general anaesthesia or nitrous oxide (laughing gas), which is quite commonly used in the US.

Therefore, local anaesthesia (which numbs only the area of operation) is the commonest option for our dentists. The drug used most frequently for this is lignocaine (other occasional alternatives are articaine and bupivacaine). As a 2 per cent concentrate, the anaesthetic is normally mixed with adrenaline to enhance and sustain its effect. This version is sometimes avoided in those with high blood pressure, or heart disease; but even cardiologists are divided in their opinion about its use.

The anaesthesia is injected with a disposable/sterilized syringe and needle. Single-use cartridges containing one dose of the drug are preferred, so that repeated drawings from a larger bottle or vial are avoided to prevent contamination.

Furthermore, to prevent bacterial contamination, many dentists have their patients rinse their mouths with an antiseptic mouthwash just before injecting the anaesthetic. A small dab of antiseptic may also be placed over the site where the injection is to be administered.

Except in the case of the lower back teeth, the anaesthetic injection is usually given close to the teeth being treated. For the lower back teeth, a major nerve at the back of the mouth needs to be numbed, so the injection is given accordingly in this area.

In modern dental clinics, the only pain that may be felt is the poke of the needle while injecting the local anaesthetic! In fact, due to the use of sharp, disposable needles, there is *barely* any pain associated with the injection, and all that one really feels is an odd sense of pressure when the anaesthetic solution enters the tissues.

You need to know that the dentist will start the treatment *only* after checking the gums with a sharp pointed instrument called a probe, to confirm the effect of the anaesthetic. While it's not mandatory, an anaesthetic gel can be applied to temporarily numb the area where the needle will be jabbed. This is most useful for kids!

The numbness begins setting in rapidly, starting with a tingling like pins-and-needles, and proceeding to a complete lack of sensation. One may feel as if the numb area is swollen— but it is just a reflection of the anaesthesia, and there is no such swelling! The numbness lasts for two to three hours, which is more then sufficient to complete most planned procedures.

General Tooth Extraction Procedures: Feeling the Pull

The general impression about a tooth extraction is that the dentist uses a pair of pliers to grab the tooth and yank it out! Modern extractions are far more refined, and designed to use more of technique, and less of brute force. A routine extraction is a fairly simple procedure for qualified and experienced dentists.

As we are aware, teeth are not 'fixed' to the jawbone: they are suspended in the jaw socket by the tough periodontal ligament. With this premise, the teeth are loosened out or luxated using a lever principle.

After confirming that the tooth has lost full sensation, the dentist starts by separating it slightly from the gums. Specially designed instruments, called elevators and luxators, are then used to loosen the tooth from its socket. Finally, with dental forceps (the 'pliers' as people know them), the tooth is rocked back and forth, and gently prised out of its housing. Since the tooth and the adjoining area is numb, one will feel no pain whatsoever, just the pressure exerted on the tooth.

After the tooth is removed, a cotton/gauze roll, shaped like a pom-pom, is placed over the empty socket; this has to be kept bitten down in place for about thirty minutes. It is done to ensure that a blood clot forms within the socket so as to prevent further bleeding. The clot is the natural 'dressing' for the wound!

The socket slowly fills in with bone, and the surface is covered over by gum tissue—six to eight weeks and the healing and closure of the socket is complete. In the usual course, the healed gums and corresponding bone would shrink further into the jaw. This could result in compromised aesthetics, and an inability to fit a replacement later, with a firm enough footing at a later stage.

Replacement teeth can be planned either immediately following tooth extractions, during the healing phase or after completion of the healing at eight weeks. Chapter Fifteen throws more light on tooth replacements.

Recently, the emphasis has shifted to maintaining the shape and density of the jawbone at the site of the tooth extraction. Socket preservation (or alveolar ridge preservation) is a procedure to reduce bone loss at the site, and to stay the shape of the bone socket.

Following the tooth extraction, a bone substitute known

as a bone graft, is placed in the socket. The graft could be mixed with 'platelet rich fibrin' (PRF), which is derived from the patient's own blood to encourage new bone formation. Finally, the socket is covered and stitched over by a layer of thin, filmy material, known as a membrane. This process is slated to become a routine feature of tooth extractions, where the emphasis is on preserving the jawbone.

Surgical Extractions: A Cut Above

Often, wisdom teeth (the third molar), the lower ones and extra teeth (supernumerary teeth) are stalled or stuck in the jawbone for lack of space to erupt. These 'impacted' teeth, unable to erupt normally, may emerge in an angular direction and get stalled in the process. Some remain within the jaw, and may prevent normal teeth from erupting.

Across the ages, our diet has changed from the raw food that our ancestors ate, to the predominantly cooked and refined fare that we eat today. This means that we don't need too many chewing teeth, and the gradual related process of evolution has ensured that our jaw size is shrinking.

The victims of this evolutionary shrinkage are our third molars (the wisdom teeth), which are the last to erupt, and end up with insufficient space in the jaw.

If they lie dormant, without any sign of infection or damage to the other teeth, it may be best to leave them alone. However, these teeth often suffer from gum infections or rot, and can affect the adjoining teeth or cause persistent irritation to the cheeks. Rarely, these impacted teeth may also develop cysts or tumours. In such instances, dentists would advise their removal.

The extraction of an impacted third molar is a minor

surgical procedure. Once the area is numbed by local anaesthesia, the dentist makes a cut in the gums and surrounding tissues near the wisdom tooth. The bone, which may be obstructing its removal, is then chipped away with special drills.

This is accompanied by a liberal flushing of the area with cold saline that cools the region and washes away the drilling debris. The coolant effect is important, as any overheating of the delicate jawbone can result in post-operative pain or delayed healing.

Next, elevators/luxators are used to loosen the tooth from the socket, and finally the errant tooth is removed; sometimes, the tooth is also cut into smaller sections to ease its removal. At the end, the area is thoroughly cleaned and stitches or sutures tied in.

Contraindications: Pulling Back

Dental extractions are planned only after a careful medical history is taken, and after establishing that any prevailing medical conditions are under proper control. While most people can undergo a dental extraction with no serious concerns, there are some exceptions:

- Extractions are not advisable in pregnant women, except in their second trimester—months four, five and six. The rest of the time, it is best avoided unless it's an emergency and cannot be postponed till after the full term of pregnancy.
- Dental extractions may be deferred if there is an active infection in the tissues surrounding the tooth, especially in the case of a visible swelling on the face. It may be

planned after the infection is contained.

- Uncontrolled hypertension (high blood pressure) can lead to heavy bleeding after an extraction. It's best to ensure that the blood pressure is normal prior to the procedure.

- People with unchecked diabetes are likely to experience delayed healing. Their blood sugar level needs to be brought within limits before any extractions.

- Heart patients take blood thinners like aspirin, which may result in excessive blood loss after the procedure. Often, their cardiologists may advise against tooth extractions or surgical procedures, till their heart condition stabilizes.

- Some patients are on long-term therapy with anti-coagulants like Warfarin to prevent internal blood clotting. They would need to discontinue the medication, in consultation with their physician, for a few days prior to and after the extraction to prevent excessive blood loss.

- People suffering from haemophilia, or from deficiency of any of the natural blood-clotting factors, are advised against procedures that can result in bleeding, unless special precautions are instituted beforehand.

- Those who have undergone radiation around the jaws should not go in for teeth extractions immediately after their treatment. It is best done prior to the radiation.

- Patients under treatment for any serious illness need to be cleared by their physicians regarding their fitness for dental extractions.

Care Following Tooth Extraction: After the Pull-out

Tooth extraction is a simple and safe procedure in recent times. At most, a mild swelling or discomfort may be felt in the area for a few days, and the dentist could prescribe simple analgesics to counter this. Often, these are needed for just a day or two!

Routine extractions rarely need antibiotic coverage, which is reserved for situations such as a persistent local infection, or in medical conditions necessitating such medication. Modern protocols for equipment hygiene and sterilization have contributed largely to this safety valve.

After an extraction, it is important for you to follow certain instructions to ensure better pain management, quick healing and no untoward complication:

- A cotton/gauze pack is placed at the site of the extracted tooth—do bite down on this to keep it there for at least thirty minutes. This exerts pressure on the wound—and importantly—stops the bleeding and allows a blood clot to form.
- During this time, apply an ice pack on your face, in the area corresponding to the removed tooth to prevent swelling and pain.
- After thirty minutes, gently remove the pack, and discard it—please don't spit it out!
- A slight oozing of blood is common after the pack is removed. Keep swallowing it down, but don't try to spit it out.
- The blood clot that forms in the wound is imperative for not only stopping the bleeding, but also to set off the healing process. Therefore, for the next twenty-four

hours, do not spit or rinse the mouth. Avoid alcohol or smoking, and do not suck in liquids through a straw. All of these could dislodge the blood clot and open up the wound.

- Be careful to not bite your lips, cheek or tongue, which may remain numb for two to three hours following the local anaesthesia. In children, the danger of a traumatic ulcer or sore setting in is greater, as they tend to repeatedly chew these areas that feel 'like rubber'!
- Take your painkiller and any other medication as advised by the dentist.
- Following the extraction, have soft foods which are easy to swallow, and at room temperature or cold. Avoid eating on the affected side for a few days, to minimize disturbance to the healing wound.
- After twenty-four hours, warm saline rinses are recommended to alleviate discomfort, and to keep the wound free of food debris.
- Following surgical extractions, medicated mouth rinses will be prescribed by the dentist to keep the area clean, rather than run the risk of loosening the stitches by the tugging of toothbrush bristles. From the day after the removal, ensure that you brush all the other teeth as usual, taking care to avoid injuring the wound.
- After a wisdom tooth surgery, your dentist will advise jaw-stretching exercises to maintain your lower jaw movements. If you resist opening your mouth fully, guarding the jaw movements instead, it might cramp up, causing a lock-jaw.
- Report any untoward symptoms, such as persistent bleeding, pain or numbness, to your dentist immediately.

Possible Complications with Tooth Extraction: Troubling Times

Occasionally, despite all due diligence from dentists and their patients, tooth extractions can cause complications. Here are the more common ones.

Persistent Bleeding

This can be scary, as the wound keeps oozing blood. Rarely, it is triggered off due to serious injury to mouth tissues during the extraction, or because of the residual effect of blood-thinning medications.

But, in the normal course, it is because of *not* adhering to the post-extraction instructions, especially with respect to spitting, and rinsing the mouth. If there is prolonged bleeding, you could try biting down on a fresh cotton swab for half-an-hour. Despite this, if the bleeding persists, then a visit to the dentist is necessary.

Persistent Pain

One of the main causes for post-operative pain is the loss of the protective blood clot from the wound, leaving behind an empty socket, called a dry socket. This could happen due to repeated rinsing or spitting after the extraction. Smokers and women using birth-control pills are also prone to dry sockets, as the blood clot tends to disintegrate. Dentists treat this by cleaning the socket of any remaining debris and applying a soothing dressing inside it, which is changed regularly over a few days. Painkillers will help, and antibiotics may also be prescribed.

Prolonged Numbness

Usually, this is a complication seen after wisdom tooth

surgery, if there is injury to the nerves. Called paraesthesia, the numbness can affect one side of the tongue, or the lip or cheek, depending on which nerve was injured. Most instances recover with time. You must inform your dentist promptly, so that suitable medication is immediately given to initiate the chances of the full recovery of nerve sensation.

Swelling

Mild swelling is expected after a tooth extraction—all said and done, a body part was removed. But, if the swelling is large and there is fever or pus discharge, it could be a sign of infection, and antibiotics may become necessary. Surgical extractions usually cause more swelling than other procedures, as the jawbone is subjected to drilling. This is anticipated, and dentists normally prescribe antibiotics and analgesics, which help greatly in decreasing the swelling.

Loosening or Loss of Adjacent Teeth

Sometimes, the tooth adjacent to the one removed either becomes loose, or may pop out of its socket. This is due to careless technique, with skilled dentists unlikely to cause such a complication.

Removal of the Wrong Tooth

While it is not impossible to remove the wrong tooth in error, such instances are usually anecdotal.

Often, it is difficult to pinpoint the painful tooth, especially if multiple teeth are damaged. There is also a high degree of 'referred pain', which means that the pain from a tooth may radiate to one or more teeth in its vicinity, making it difficult to identify the offender. This is the usual culprit in allegations of the wrong tooth being pulled out. Careful examination and diagnosis by dentists can always save the wrong tooth from being extracted—the rest is just folklore!

Tooth extractions are universally disliked, but they form an important element of dental treatment. With today's refined techniques and superior anaesthetic drugs, a tooth extraction no longer qualifies for an alarming experience, as it has joined the ranks of safe, painless procedures.

Chapter 15

Tooth Replacement:
An Eye for an Eye, a Tooth for a Tooth

1500 BC. Take a piece of gold wire. Collect some human teeth, by whichever means appeals to you. Thread one of these with the wire. Ask your patient to keep his mouth open. Fasten the threaded tooth into the gap of his missing tooth. Secure it tightly to the adjacent teeth. Present your bill.

This could well be an excerpt from a dentist's work manual in ancient Egypt, as archaeologists have unearthed evidence of such tooth replacements! Proof of artificial substitutes for lost teeth has been found in several earlier civilizations. From animal teeth (Etruscans, 700 BC), to seashell and bone teeth (Mayans, 600 AD), to wooden teeth (Japan, 1500 AD), humans have been experimenting with every possible option for tooth substitutes.

This underscores the fact that even ancient peoples realized the importance of teeth. Yet, today, there are many who still prefer to be gap-toothed!

The Problems Associated with Missing Teeth: Falling Through the Gaps

Teeth—as much as any of our body parts—are fundamental to our overall functioning. Just as the little finger has its task cut out in the workings of the hand, *each tooth* has its own job to do as well. This means that when even one tooth is missing, it affects the efficiency of the other teeth, because they all perform as a unit.

A wheel can continue to roll even if a couple of spokes are missing, but without any assurance of reliability. As the load on the remaining spokes increases, they will bend or break, further weakening the wheel. The same goes for our teeth, and missing teeth can prove to be a spoke in the wheel, gradually crippling the system in many ways.

For one, chewing gets more difficult, as teeth do not mesh together. Digestion is obviously affected when the food is not chewed well. The joint between the jaws, the temporomandibular joint, also suffers damage because of the trauma caused by the abnormal chewing positions of the teeth. Moreover, the adjacent *and* opposing teeth migrate into the gaps, losing contact with their neighbours. This leads to food getting jammed in these narrow spaces forming between the teeth, creating gum problems and cavities.

The missing tooth causes an extra load on the other teeth, subjecting them to excessive wear and tear, and compromising their function and strength over time. Speech gets altered, as teeth have a strong impact on clear diction.

The shape of the face changes, due to the lack of support from the teeth to the facial muscles. Also, missing teeth are deemed as unsightly—this can affect a person's self-esteem considerably. Besides, gaps in the front teeth can cause embarrassment, especially when saliva escapes from the mouth while speaking.

Dentists offer a wide range of options to replace missing teeth—from low-cost temporary dentures, to high-tech dental implants. Replacements are possible for one or more teeth, or even when all the teeth are missing. Some of these are removable by the wearer; others are permanently fixed in place. Let's have a look at the various types of tooth surrogates.

Removable Dentures: A Denture in Hand Is Worth...

Removable artificial teeth, which replace one or more missing ones, are known as removable partial dentures (RPD). If all the teeth are missing, complete dentures replace a full set of twenty-eight teeth (wisdom teeth aren't replaced!).

Both partial and complete dentures comprise a 'fitting' component known as a 'base', onto which artificial teeth are attached. Early forms of the base used ivory or porcelain, which were hard and unyielding. Obviously, these were also expensive and out of reach for the common man. Teeth, used as proxies, were from other mammals like cows, horses and donkeys.

Sometimes, bones from other animals, shells or ivory were attached. Human teeth were used whenever available, but they were scarce. In 1815, nearly 50,000 young British soldiers died in the battle of Waterloo, and grisly as it may sound, their teeth were harvested for use in dentures. These 'Waterloo dentures' were affordable, because of the plentiful supply at the dentists' disposal.

In the 1850s, Goodyear (of tyre fame) developed a material known as vulcanite, a form of hardened rubber, which could also be moulded into shape as a well-fitting base! Porcelain teeth could be fixed to it, and these vulcanite dentures were popular for decades.

Today, acrylic resins are in vogue for the denture base, and some removable versions are made with metal bases as well. The teeth for these are also of tough acrylic, and occasionally porcelain. Acrylic is cheaper and kinder to the temporomandibular joint, but doesn't last as long as the more aesthetic and tougher porcelain option.

Removable Partial Dentures (RPD)

These are made with acrylic, metal, or flexible resin bases. Partial dentures fit around the existing teeth, to which they are anchored by extensions, known as clasps.

To create removable partial dentures, the dentist takes an impression of both the jaws. The impression material is then loaded onto a carrying device, known as an impression tray, and placed in the mouth till it sets. This produces the negative mould, into which a substance similar to plaster-of-paris—dental stone—is poured. The stone sets hard, producing a positive replica of the teeth and gums, known as a model.

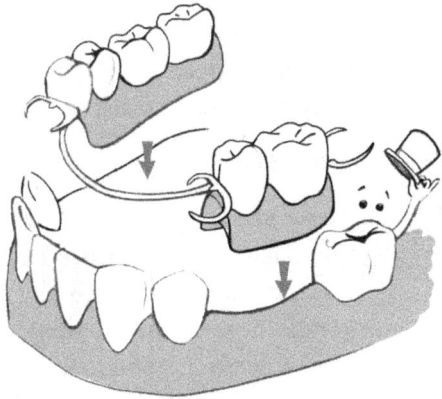

The model is sent to the dental laboratory, which manufactures the denture. The dentist may need to complete a couple of trials during the initial stages of its fabrication, which helps guide the laboratory to ensure a perfect fit, good aesthetics and proper functioning.

There are a range of options available for such dentures.

Acrylic Base RPD

These dentures are favoured, and fairly inexpensive. The base is formed of a resin, known as PMMA (or polymethyl methacrylate). Metal clasps, made of thick steel wire, are embedded in the acrylic denture, and which grasp the adjacent teeth to keep the denture in place.

This is a good option for temporary or provisional usage, not for the long-term. The acrylic resin is porous, and hosts heaps of bacteria—a fertile ground for the spoilage of those teeth over which the denture rests. Allergic reactions to the resin are also common, and sometimes, the metal clasps can wear away the enamel of the clasped teeth.

Unfortunately, acrylic RPDs tend to be used for too long by wearers, leading to significant damage to the other natural teeth they rest against.

Metal Base RPD

These use a custom cast metal base, which also incorporates the clasps. An alloy of cobalt and chrome is preferred for this, as it is strong and totally corrosion-free. A gum-coloured acrylic is used in the areas of the missing teeth, to which acrylic teeth are bonded.

These dentures are remarkably strong and durable, and the minimized contact between the acrylic parts and the natural teeth prevents decay.

The flip side is that the metallic clasps can look unseemly. Also, these dentures require minor shaping of the natural teeth, to ensure a correct fit and proper transfer of load to the supporting ones.

Flexible Dentures

Currently, flexible polymers are also available for this denture base, which can be gum-coloured, or even clear. Known as thermoplastic resins, usually with a nylon component, some of the popular materials in this category include Valplast™,

Flexiplast™ and Flexite™. Being strong and malleable, they can be used to form the clasps too, thus totally avoiding the use of metal.

The aesthetics, therefore, are excellent! There are several other positives. Unlike acrylic resins, these have virtually no porosity, offering little opportunity for bacterial accumulation on their surface. They are virtually unbreakable, and unlike metal dentures, the natural teeth need no shaping or preparation. They can be fabricated in a short time, giving you reasonably quick replacements. As they are removable, they are easy to clean as well. They are also relatively inexpensive when compared to fixed replacements.

★

Once the dentist receives the customized denture, it is checked for imperfections, if any. Then, he fits it in your mouth and checks if it fixes correctly. The appearance and 'bite' contact of the denture are also inspected, and adjustments made as necessary.

When all parameters are satisfactory, the dentist demonstrates to you the right manner in which the denture is to be placed in your mouth. It is best if you try it on yourself, under the supervision of the dentist, to ensure that you get it right. You are now ready to flash your new pearlies!

A few follow up visits may be necessary for the dentist to attend to trouble spots, or areas of discomfort; the dentures may need to be loosened or tightened. Removable dentures do have an adaptation period, and it could take a few days for them to settle down into a good functioning mode. With a little perseverance, they will serve to their optimum potential.

However, removable partial dentures are not very popular, as they come with their own set of problems:

- They tend to be bulky, leaving a foreign body sensation in the mouth.
- The need to wear and remove them everyday can be a nuisance.
- During meals, food particles tend to get under the dentures, creating irritation. It may become necessary to remove them for cleaning after every meal.
- Loosening or dislodgement of the denture while speaking and eating can be acutely embarrassing in public.
- Chewing efficiency with RPDs is not as good as with fixed teeth.
- Speech can be affected—pronunciation of sibilants and certain words is difficult, especially with dentures that replace the front teeth.
- The need to keep the dentures in water when not in use is often forgotten. If not stored securely, they can get misplaced too.
- Needing to clean the denture thoroughly is an added chore. If its fitting surface is not kept clean, it can lead to bacterial overgrowth, or cause fungal infections of the mouth tissues it rests on.
- Unclean dentures can promote cavity formation in the natural teeth on which they rest.
- Removable partial dentures, especially small ones, can get inadvertently swallowed. If these are very loose, there is a choking hazard too.
- Dentures that replace the last few teeth with no supporting tooth behind them can induce pain in the soft tissues.
- The clasps of RPDs can exert excessive force on the supporting teeth that they hold on to, weakening them

in the process.

- With flexible dentures, It could be difficult for the dentist to smoothen and polish any adjustments made during the fitting. They are also expensive and tend to get stained by food colours.

Considering all these shortcomings, it is important to be mentally accepting of them—otherwise, there is a tendency to avoid wearing them altogether, and they remain in the box!

Removable Complete Dentures (RCD)

Our teeth are designed to last a lifetime, just like any other body part. It is indeed a myth that our teeth will inevitably get loose and fall off as we age. Unless they are knocked out in an accident, most teeth that are lost are due to disease caused by neglect!

When teeth are completely mutilated, they have to be extracted. A total decimation of the teeth is usually the result of extensive breakdown due to dental caries, or advanced gum disorder. In the case of the latter, most teeth may simply fall off, and the rest too loose to be saved by treatment.

A complete denture is needed in such cases—for those who have no teeth at all! It is the last resort, when all treatment options to preserve the natural teeth are exhausted. Many people feel that it is a great alternative to going through

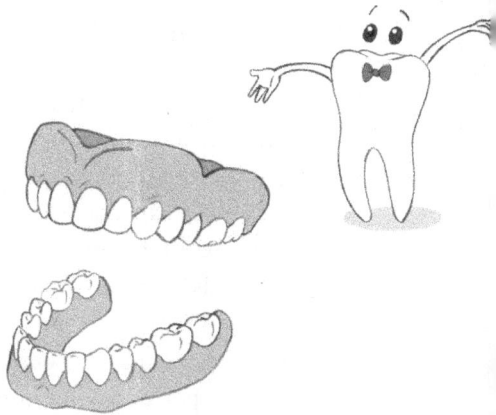

extensive and expensive dental treatment to save the teeth. This couldn't be further from the truth! Even a well-made complete denture is just a poor substitute for our natural teeth, attaining only 20 per cent of their chewing ability!

After all the teeth are extracted or lost, it takes nearly three months for the bone and gums to heal. Since that area shrinks and changes its shape through this period, the final dentures are best made after healing is complete. Most people find it extremely punishing to manage the three-month interim without teeth—so temporary dentures or 'immediate dentures' are the norm today.

Immediate Complete Dentures

Waiting for dentures after losing all your teeth can seem interminable! Without them, eating and chewing are obviously affected, but the impact on appearance and speech is worse. The facial structure collapses without tooth support, and all of a sudden, the person looks twenty years older. Speech becomes garbled, and can affect communication. With no teeth to guide their movements, the jaws lose their orientation to each other—this can make it terribly hard to adjust later to the chewing relationship of new dentures.

To avoid this serious handicap, dentists recommend using immediate dentures, which can be readied prior to the extractions. The jaws are measured, their replicas created and mock extractions performed on them. The laboratory creates the complete denture based on this dummy, which closely resembles the shape the jaws would actually assume after the teeth are extracted. This immediate denture is placed in the mouth on the day the last of the teeth are removed.

These dentures fit reasonably well, but as the wounds heal with time, they get loose. This may necessitate a denture adhesive, a gum-like paste, which helps to keep it in place. With its help, the facial appearance is virtually unchanged, and though speech may be affected initially, it quickly clears up.

While a soft diet is recommended in the early days, one can start chewing on food, gently, within a couple of weeks. This not only allows the jaws to adapt to the new chewing technique, it also aids the digestive process.

Final Complete Dentures

Around six weeks after extraction of all the teeth, the gums and the underlying bone support can be examined for their readiness to provide a reasonable fitting for a new denture. Occasionally, sharp bony projections or irregular contours may remain, which would need to be smoothened via a minor surgical procedure, under local anaesthesia. When the healing is complete, at around three months, the final dentures can be made.

As with removable partial dentures, the base for complete dentures can be made of metal, acrylic or flexible resins. Similarly, the artificial teeth can be of acrylic or porcelain.

There are several sequential steps in the making of complete dentures:

1. Impressions
The fit of the denture depends on how accurately the shape of the healed gums can be recorded. For this purpose, dentists make precise impressions using materials that capture the fine details with great fidelity. These impressions are negative replicas of the shape of the denture-supporting portion of the mouth.

2. Jaw Relation
The dentist needs to record the exact manner in which the

upper and lower jaws meet each other. Known as 'jaw relation', it helps in setting the artificial teeth into the correct alignment, and in the right chewing or 'bite' relationship.

3. Try-in

A mock set-up of the proposed arrangement of teeth in the denture is tried on in the mouth. The look, as well as good functional interlocking of the upper and lower artificial teeth, are established.

Ideally, it would be great if a family member or friend could accompany the proposed wearer, to endorse the new look of the artificial teeth. Any changes found necessary can be accommodated at this stage, by repositioning the teeth to suit the individual's face, within the existing parameters. Once both dentist and patient approve the trial set-up, the model is sent to the lab for the final assembly.

4. Denture Delivery

When the finished denture comes from the lab, the dentist inserts it into the patient's mouth to check for any adjustments that may be needed in refining its fit and chewing positions. Once everything's approved, it's time for the wearer to beam the falsies!

Overdentures

In the absence of all the teeth, the jawbone shrinks continuously (and at a faster pace in the case of diabetics, and post-menopausal women). In denture-wearers, this leads to an increasingly loose fit.

To help resolve this issue, and if the situation permits, it may be possible to retain a couple of teeth in each jaw, usually the canines. They are given root canal treatment, and trimmed down to small stubs, so that the complete dentures can be fashioned to fit over, and fully cover them. These teeth act not only as pillars for better grounding of the overdentures, they also preserve the height of the bone in these two areas. Many users report an easier chewing experience, thanks to them.

If the retained teeth are really sound, overdentures can be further improved by adding 'precision attachments'. One option is in the form of a ball, attached to the retained tooth, which fits into a dedicated socket on the underside of the denture. Another variant is a metal bar connecting the two retained teeth, with special clips on the underside of the denture clamped to the bar.

★

Complete dentures stay in place due to a close fit—the thin film of saliva between the denture and the gums creating the holding force, known as capillary action. (The same force causes plastic coasters to stick to the bottom of a glass of water, when lifted!) This hold is stronger in the upper dentures, as the area under coverage is larger, on account of the palate. Therefore, upper dentures stay well in place, unless there is violent coughing or sneezing. In the lower dentures, a much narrower horseshoe shaped area is available to hold them, since the tongue needs to be given ample room for movement. As a result, lower dentures are prone to coming loose easily.

Over time, wearers adapt to their dentures—the muscles of the lips, inner cheeks and tongue needing time to accept their presence. Eventually, the entire team starts working in tandem, preventing the denture from getting loose when speaking or chewing.

New wearers need to keep the denture on for a few hours every day, and increase the duration of wear gradually. Chewing with dentures also takes time to get familiar with, as they can get skewed if you chew from only one side. Unlike our natural teeth, these artificial ones are interconnected via the base, creating a seesaw effect by raising the denture from the unused side. The need to chew in a balanced way, on both sides simultaneously needs to be learnt.

In the early days, it is best to stick to eating softer foods, as this minimizes the chances of injury. As the denture settles in and becomes comfortable, chewing firmer foods can be attempted.

Since the jawbone continues to shrink under complete dentures, their fit worsens. Most dentures may need their fitting bases to be altered, or even remade once in three or four years.

Good home care of dentures is a must, as it keeps them working well over the years. A few guidelines follow:

- They must be removed at night, and put away—this gives your teeth and gums a much-needed breather. The mouth tends to dry out during the night, which can affect the fit of some dentures.
- Soak the dentures in water overnight—because if they dry out, they could crack, or change shape.
- Your dentures need to be cleaned well twice a day— remove them from the mouth so that you can get at all the surfaces. A stiff toothbrush is efficacious for this, together with mild soap (toothpastes could abrade the surface polish of the dentures). You must rinse off all the soap after use.
- Occasionally, dentures can slip out of your hands while washing, leading to breakage. This can be prevented by cleaning them inside the washbasin in which a soft towel is placed to cushion any falls. In case the denture

does break, it can, more often than not, be repaired at a dental laboratory.

- Although none are as superior to a daily scrubbing with soap, commercial products are also available for cleaning dentures, in the form of a paste, or as tablets that bubble up when added to water.
- Your dentures may merit special instructions, which your dentist can best explain—follow these, as everyone's dentures are unique!

With good maintenance, removable dentures can serve well for around four to five years, after which changes in the supporting tissues of the mouth, coupled with normal wear and tear, may necessitate their replacement.

Fixed Partial Dentures: Building Bridges

A fixed partial denture, popularly known as a 'bridge', solves one of the biggest drawbacks of an RPD—it is a permanent fixture!

Bridges take the support of adjacent natural teeth, and quickly blend in: over time, many people actually forget that they have a bridge fixed in their mouth!

The primary requirement for this option is the presence of healthy, strong teeth ahead of and behind the missing tooth/teeth. Your dentist can recommend a bridge only if these supporting teeth are deemed capable of taking on the load.

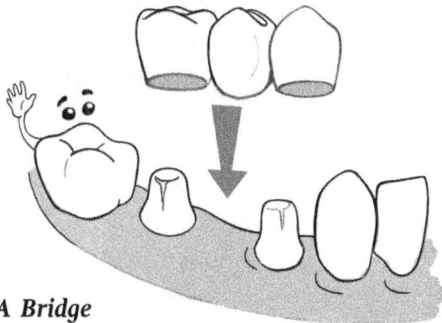

A Bridge

Fixing Bridges

A bridge essentially comprises a crown or cap, on each of the supporting teeth, between which the artificial teeth are attached. In tech-speak, the prepared supporting teeth are called 'abutments', the crowns fixed over them are called 'retainers' and the component of artificial teeth is known as a 'pontic'.

The preparation of the supporting teeth is identical to that of crowning a tooth (described in Chapter Thirteen). The supporting teeth are ground down to a smaller specific shape to receive the retainers. As with the crowning process, high-speed drills are used until the teeth look like miniature versions of themselves. While sculpting the desired shape, the dentist also provides an accurate margin or step, on which the edges of the retainer will eventually sit.

Many dentists advise a preventive endodontic or root canal treatment for the supporting teeth, as the preparation process can bring their dental pulp closer to the surface, and even breach it occasionally.

If this is not done, a bridge over such teeth would lead to constant sensitivity and pain, and the pulp could die out gradually, causing an infection. Access for performing the necessary root canal treatment now becomes difficult once the bridge is fixed on—a hole would need to be drilled through it to reach the damaged pulp! Therefore, wherever it is anticipated, it is prudent to carry out such pre-emptive endodontic treatment.

Once the tooth is prepared and ready, an accurate impression is taken to create a replica of the teeth, known as a model or cast. This goes away to a dental laboratory, which fabricates the bridge in the next few days.

In the interim, dentists put in place a temporary bridge, which occupies and preserves the space for the final one. Made of tooth-coloured resin, it is designed for short-term use, so its looks and function may not be as good as that of the final bridge. Most dentists assemble these immediately after the impressions for the bridge are completed, and fix them in the jaws with temporary cements, enabling their easy removal when needed.

Composition of Bridges

Dental laboratories use the same materials for bridges as for crowns. Let's look at the composition of bridges:

- Bridges can be made entirely of metal, such as nickel-chromium alloy, or even with alloys of precious metals like gold, palladium, etc. Laboratories use a casting process, employing a lost-wax technique, to create metal and metal-based bridges.
- Tooth-coloured bridges are crafted by covering metal cores with a coating of porcelain (ceramic) or resin. These are known as PFM or porcelain-fused-to-metal-bridges.
- Some ceramic materials are available in high-strength versions (for instance, Empress™), in which metal cores can be avoided for better looks. These are useful in low-stress areas, as in the front teeth.
- Recent developments include metal-free bridges, in which zirconia—a white, rugged material of very high strength—replaces the metallic core. They can be used for the back teeth as well, due to their toughness.
- High-strength bridges, made entirely of zirconia, are also now available.

Bridge Innovations

We now also have crowns and bridges created by CAD-CAM technology—a computerized production using a 3D image of the prepared, trimmed teeth. And, still rolling off the shelf are cutting-edge solutions called chair-side CAD/CAM. Here, the dentist takes a 3D image of the prepared teeth with a scanning device, which is then sent to a computerised milling machine. Using ceramic or metal ingots and milling burs, the crown/bridge is produced rapidly in this machine, and can be fitted on the very same day.

Another type of fixed bridge—preferred for the replacement of a single missing front tooth—and which tries to minimize the shaping of supporting teeth, is known as a resin-retained bridge. (One of the popular designs is called the Maryland bridge.) In this procedure, the supporting teeth are reduced just a bit on their tongue-facing surfaces, not going deeper than the enamel layer. The laboratory fabricates the bridge, whose artificial tooth has metallic wing-like extensions on either side, which fit precisely into these prepared surfaces of the supporting teeth. The biggest advantage of this bridge is the reduced miniaturization of healthy teeth, but this could, conversely, lead to a compromise in the retention of the bridge itself. It can get unbonded or dislodged, which could prove to be embarrassing and inconvenient.

Getting the Best Out of a Bridge

Irrespective of the method of fabrication, when the finished bridge is received, the temporary one is removed. The dentist first checks the fit, shape and colour-match of the bridge. Next, its contacts with neighbouring and opposing teeth are verified. Then it is permanently fixed into place using strong dental cements. Voila! It is done!

Here are a few tips on getting the best out of your new bridge:

- You would do well to avoid chewing on it the day it is installed.
- Over the next few days, the bridge might feel a bit odd due to the 'newness' factor. However, this settles down quickly, and it soon feels like a part of the mouth.
- Maintain meticulous hygiene around the bridge, including daily flossing.
- Over the long term, avoid subjecting it to very sticky foods, such as chocolate éclairs, chewy candy, chikki, etc. These can exert a pull-away force, and may cause the bridge to come undone.
- If your bridge feels loose, or seems to have changed position, or even comes off totally, please see your dentist immediately. A loose bridge can be re-fixed without incident, as long as it's done without delay. Otherwise, it may not fit into place accurately due to the subtle movements of the supporting and/or opposing teeth.
- Avoid biting on very hard food with ceramic or ceramic-coated bridges: ceramics are hard, but brittle, and could chip off, exposing the unsightly metal underneath.

The Pros and Cons of Bridges

Structurally, bridges are fairly strong and durable, and can last several years. The weak link is usually the supporting teeth underneath: failed bridges are often on account of the breakdown of supports due to decay.

Fixed bridges score over removable dentures on various counts:

- The nuisance of removing and cleaning a denture is totally avoided.
- The replacement is in line with the other teeth, and doesn't feel bulky or foreign.
- The fixed artificial tooth can take a stronger chewing load, and needs to be cleaned much like any of the other natural teeth.

However, there are a few areas of concern:

- Bridges are usually more expensive than removable dentures.
- One of the main drawbacks is that natural teeth adjacent to the missing one need to be trimmed down to accommodate the fixed bridge. This can necessitate further interventions on the supporting teeth, such as root canal treatment, to prevent them from turning sensitive or painful.
- In metal-based bridges, grey shadows may be visible along the gum line due to the show-through of the metal.
- An extra step is added to the usual oral hygiene routine—the need to floss under the bridge, where the artificial tooth contacts the gums. This is done with a floss-threader, a plastic needle-like device to carry the floss under the pontic.
- If the supporting teeth are not strong enough, they could weaken under the extra load, and suffer damage.
- Poor oral hygiene around bridges can expose the supporting teeth to decay and gum disease.

Having said this, fixed bridges have an expected lifespan exceeding ten years. Many factors influence its longevity, including oral hygiene, chewing habits, decay or gum disease, etc. Regular professional attention can enhance its life, keeping you smiling for years!

Chapter 16

Dental Implants: Feel It in Your Bones

Imagine an artificial tooth, which is firmly fixed inside the jawbone and can't develop cavities. Welcome to the world of dental implants! Going way beyond conventional means of tooth replacement, these are designed to closely mimic the way natural teeth stay rooted in place.

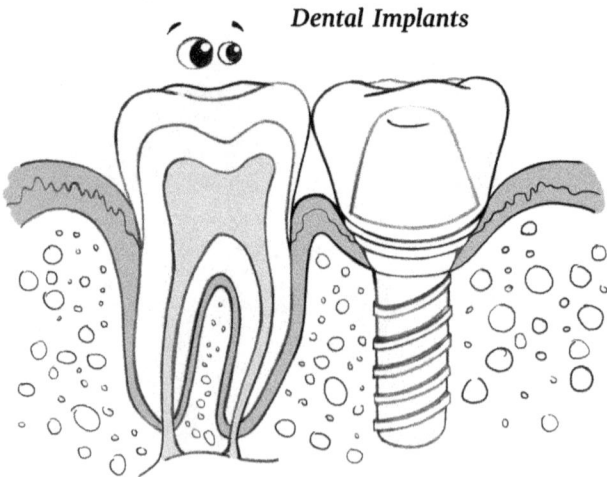

Dental Implants

Humans have experimented with such restorations for many thousands of years. Egyptian archaeologists found evidence of a shell fixed inside the jaw of a mummy, which could well have been a dental implant! However, there is no conclusive evidence of whether it was a ceremonial ornament related to the burial process instead, or was indeed functional during the life of the person.

One of the remains from the great Mayan civilization, around 600 AD, shows three shells implanted in a recovered jaw, which seem to have fused with the bone. They were subjected to considerable use in the person's lifetime—with tartar deposits on them!

Dental implants, as we know them now in the modern world, came about only after 1950. Swedish orthopaedic surgeon, Dr Brånemark, was engaged in research at Cambridge University, during which time he serendipitously came across an amazing occurrence. He had inserted tiny titanium cylinders into the bones of rabbits as an experiment, and found that he couldn't remove them when he needed to. They had completely fused with the bone!

This exciting find compelled further research, and the conclusion was inescapable: under the right conditions, a titanium screw inserted into the jawbone encourages the bone to grow around it and lock it in place. This phenomenon has been called 'osseointegration'—in other words, becoming one with bone. It is the basic principle on which different types of dental implants have been developed.

When Implants Are Recommended: Setting Your Teeth on Edge

Titanium is the preferred choice of metal for an implant, as it is considered the most compatible with our oral tissues and jawbone. Usually in the form of a thick screw, which is inserted into the jawbone, it gradually fuses with the bone.

The union is secure, and can easily take normal chewing loads.

Here are the typical situations where implants can be used:

- To replace a single missing tooth
- In larger gaps, two implants can support a bridge
- In certain cases, when multiple implants can serve as supports to hold fixed bridges replacing all the teeth in a jaw
- When multiple implants can permanently fix a complete denture
- When two or more implants can become the supports for an overdenture (this accords better stability to loose dentures)

The Ideal Time for Implants: Let's Sink Our Teeth into This

So, when is the best time to get yourself a dental implant? There are three time windows for this.

Immediately Following a Tooth Extraction

Here, the empty socket is suitably prepared, and the implant is inserted into it. To ensure success, the extraction needs to be done cleanly, and there should be no extensive infection in the tooth.

Around Four to Six Weeks Following a Tooth Extraction

At this stage, the wound is filled with healing tissue, making it favourable for receiving an implant.

After the Socket of the Extracted Tooth Has Completely Healed

This happens at around three months—the healing is over,

but there's the possibility of some loss of bone density and volume.

There are two major components of successful implant treatment:

- The actual insertion of the implant in the jawbone—a surgical procedure
- The construction of the functional tooth over the implant—the restorative or prosthetic phase

In the original treatment protocol recommended by Dr Brånemark, this final restoration or replacement would be carried out after a period of three to six months. The wait would allow the implant to firm up completely in the bone, and only after confirming this would the tooth be put into place.

Today, with improvements in implant design and techniques, and based on the quality of the jawbone, the tooth replacement can be fixed immediately after the implant insertion (termed 'immediate loading') or within two months (called 'early loading').

The Process of Implanting Teeth: Turning the Screws

The key to a successful implant is planning it right. First, the medical history of the recipient needs to be clear; then the dentist makes a comprehensive evaluation of the jaws and teeth. The quality and quantity of the bone at the site are crucial factors that need to be determined. Apart from this, the dentist also checks out the local conditions, the gums and neighbouring tissues, the opposing teeth, etc.

To achieve a thorough evaluation, the dentist conducts a detailed physical examination of the mouth. A CT (computerized tomography) scan, and individual X-rays of the area and of the entire jaw are some of the diagnostics the dentist relies on. In addition, impressions of the jaws are also taken for study. The number of implants needed, their ideal locations, and their correct size can be ascertained after all this data is analysed.

The insertion of the implants is conducted under a strict, germ-free surgical protocol. Initially, a local anaesthetic is used to numb the area. Next, a small cut is made in the gums to expose the jawbone at the site of the proposed implant (alternately, gum tissue is removed, wherever possible, through a small keyhole opening).

Specialized high-power slow speed drills are used to carve out a precise hole in the bone, whose size corresponds exactly to that of the implant. The drilling is accomplished with plenty of cool water or saline to prevent heat damage to the delicate jawbone. Prefabricated guides, known as surgical stents, steer the precise placement of the implants.

Artificial bone substitute, known as bone graft, may be necessitated to shore up the possibility of insufficient jawbone. This is especially so when the implant is being inserted immediately after a tooth extraction—but can also be applied in all instances of any inadequacy of available bone. Other surgical procedures to accommodate the implant could be needed concomitantly, such as raising the floor of the nasal sinus (known as a 'sinus lift'), or relocating the nerve within the lower jaw (known as 'inferior alveolar nerve repositioning').

The implants are placed in the dedicated drilled holes, either by manually screwing them in, or with an electrical drill to thread them in. Some implants can even be gently tapped into place.

If the restoration is to be delayed, the implant is buried

within and the gums stitched over it. In case a keyhole procedure is followed, a small stud-like attachment (called a 'healing abutment') is placed over the implant, which projects from the gum line. (See the next section for an explanation of abutments.)

If immediate restorations or replacements have been pre-planned, these are placed immediately or within forty-eight hours. In other cases, the implant is allowed to heal for three to six months.

After the firm union of the implant with the bone is established through X-rays and physical evaluation, the replacement phase can begin. A small surgery exposes the implant that was buried under the gums, and the healing abutment is fixed. (This is a small stud-like device which projects into the mouth, allowing the gums to heal around the implant.)

Post-Implant Instructions: Down in the Mouth

After the surgery, your dentist will, most likely, leave you with these instructions:

- Avoid eating from the operated side in the early days. If you've had multiple implants inserted, stick to items that can be swallowed, like soft and cold foods, or liquids.
- Avoid alcohol on the day of the procedure. Smoking will delay healing, and is best curtailed for at least two months.
- Some swelling and pain could result on account of the surgery. Mild analgesics and antibiotics may be prescribed, and need to be taken accordingly.

- If stitches are incorporated, toothbrushing is to be avoided at the site; mouthwashes are therefore recommended for several days after surgery to keep the area clean.
- Hard, heavy foods are best avoided on the implanted area during the healing period.

Abutments: Give It Some Teeth

The healing abutment, when used, allows the gum tissues to develop and adapt properly around it, forming a collar. When it is removed, another component is screwed into the implant, known as an implant abutment—a reduced tooth, over which a crown, bridge, or complete denture can be fitted.

When immediate replacements are planned, the implant abutment is instantly screwed into the implant. Very often, especially in the case of the front teeth, the implant may be fixed straightaway, with a temporary crown for aesthetic reasons. Indeed, some manufacturers offer a composite 'one-piece' implant and abutment combination, suitable for prompt replacements. Abutments are also available in tooth-coloured options for aesthetically crucial areas.

When a single implant is inserted for replacing one tooth, the abutment is fitted, and impressions made for a crown. This can then be fixed, either with cement as per custom, or directly to the implant with a screw.

A similar process is followed when two or more implants are placed to support a bridge.

When a fixed complete denture is planned using implants, multiple implants are inserted into the jaw. Their individual abutments are joined to each other with a titanium bar, creating a framework. This framework is embedded into the fitting portion of the complete denture, and fixed into each implant with screws.

When removable complete dentures need additional support, implant-supported overdentures are hugely effective. Two to four implants can be inserted in a jaw and overlaid with ball-shaped abutments, which fit into sockets on the underside of the denture. Alternately, a metal bar is placed, which connects the implants, and clips inserted on the underside of the denture latch on to this bar, improving the stability of the denture.

Assessing Implants: While Comparisons Are Odious...

Dental implants are the rage today, as they score over other more traditional forms of tooth replacement, quite remarkably. Let's see how they compare with the conventional options:

Implants Versus Conventional Complete Dentures

When a removable complete denture is supported by implants (that is, an implant-supported overdenture), it is more stable, with less likelihood of slipping or jumping out of the mouth—avoiding inconvenience and embarrassment. The added stability significantly improves the chewing function and speech. Users can enjoy all their favourite foods!

On the other hand, when a complete denture is *fixed* to multiple implants in the jaw, it is often like a dream-come-true! The dentures don't need to be removed at all! The dentures are firm and solid through all the normal activities and they don't loosen over time. They don't shift, even during fits of coughing or sneezing, which tend to dislodge removable dentures!

Thanks to the greater retention and stability factor, using

implants to support or fix complete dentures greatly enhances the confidence levels of wearers.

Implants Versus Conventional Bridges

The single most important advantage of a replaced tooth held by an implant is the fact that the supporting teeth don't need to be trimmed. Left untouched, this helps avoid additional interventions like root canal treatment for the latter.

With firmer anchorage, the implanted tooth or bridge contributes a more satisfactory chewing ability. The stability and longevity of the adjacent teeth are not compromised, as they are not lending any of their strength to the artificial tooth.

There is very little maintenance required to keep the implant clean and hygienic. While natural teeth that support a bridge can decay, implants never do!

Implants, Drawbacks and Contraindications: Watch Your Mouth!

The fact that removable partial dentures and complete dentures are still in extensive use, indicates that there are limitations and drawbacks to dental implants.

The overriding reason for patients not opting for dental implants is the cost factor. Implant-based teeth, bridges and dentures, are much dearer than their traditional alternatives.

Besides, implant treatment can be time consuming. Often, there are multiple stages, such as tooth extraction, implant insertion, final replacement, etc., which need several sittings. In addition, there are long intervals between the stages.

Finally, this therapy cannot be planned in the absence of favourable circumstances. While dental implants have revolutionized the replacement of missing teeth, not everyone is a suitable candidate for it. Numerous factors need to be in sync:

- Those who receive implants should be in good general health, so as to support the healing process. This rules out patients on steroids, with active malignancies, etc.
- The quality and quantity of the jawbone for the implants must match up to the required standards. Alternatively, conditions to augment these via bone grafting ought to be feasible.
- Implants are avoided in youngsters whose bones are still developing.
- Pregnancy is obviously a bad time to perform dental implants.
- Dental implants may not be able to tolerate the heavy pressures of tooth-grinding (bruxism) and clenching of teeth. Thus, victims of these habits are out of the reckoning for such therapy.
- Diabetics are not ideal candidates for dental implants, and in those with poor control of their sugar levels, implants are avoided altogether.
- Chronic smokers are at high risk of implant rejection—they need to quit at least a couple of months prior to, and after, the operation, for a more successful outcome.
- Alcoholics may show poor compliance towards care instructions, and this can lead to failed implants. The same is true in everyone with substance-abuse issues.
- The jawbone cannot tolerate any surgical procedure in patients undergoing bisphosphonate therapy for brittle bones (osteoporosis), or who have received radiation to the jaws for cancer treatment.
- Individuals who are unmotivated about oral hygiene are not considered good candidates for implants.

Though one doesn't need to go overboard to maintain implant-supported replacements, it is still necessary to care for them as one would the natural teeth. Brushing and flossing are musts, as are regular follow-up visits. Gum disease is known to occur around implants, and professional scaling is needed for them, too.

What also makes people pause before considering dental implants are the complications that could be associated with such therapy:

- As surgical procedures are involved, issues such as infection and bleeding may arise.
- Damage to the nerves in the lower jaw can occur, leading to prolonged numbness. Implants in the upper jaw could breach the sinus of the nose, leading to sinus infection.
- Implants may not fuse with the jawbone for certain reasons, and might need to be removed.
- If not well maintained, implants can develop a condition similar to gum disease, known as 'peri-implantitis', which could break down the union between the implant and bone.

Having said that, the dental implant is the closest option to a natural tooth, when it comes to form *and* function. Today, implant therapy has become safe and predictable, and is becoming increasingly affordable too. Successful implants can keep you munching away and smiling for years!

Chapter 17

Orthodontics: Get It Straight

It's a warm, sunny day in 3000 BC. A young Egyptian boy walks into his doctor's office, and wants his crooked teeth evened out. The good ol' doc uses a wire made of catgut (derived from sheep's intestines), and wraps it around his patient's teeth. A little tweak here and there, and he's done. Having had his first taste of orthodontic treatment, his patient goes back home with mummy.

The desire for having well-aligned teeth is not new! Attempts at getting them to fall in line have been made by man for aeons, proof of this fact cropping up regularly. Greeks, Etruscans, Romans—nearly every major civilization has left signs of their efforts at creating well-ordered teeth.

Gold and silver wires were the mainstay of early experiments at orthodontics, but the modern avatar in stainless steel developed rapidly in the twentieth century. Becoming popular in the 1960s, it made orthodontic treatment more affordable and simpler.

From the metallic smiles of the 1970s to the near invisible braces of the twenty-first century, the field of orthodontics has come a long way!

Kinds of Misaligned Teeth: Out of Line

Perfectly aligned teeth add plenty of charm to the smile! Not only do they look good, but they also work efficiently, blending the best of form and function.

Unfortunately, teeth don't always erupt in a straight line. When the upper and lower teeth don't meet each other in the right manner while chewing, it is known as a bad bite or a malocclusion. There are many different forms of misalignment such as:

- Protruded upper teeth (or increased 'overjet')
- Upper front teeth that bite down too much over the lower front teeth (or increased 'overbite')
- When the upper and lower front teeth don't overlap at all (or 'open bite') when the back teeth meet.
- When the lower front teeth overlap the upper front teeth (or 'cross bite')
- When there are large gaps between adjacent teeth (or 'spacing')
- Where adjacent teeth are bunched up against each other (or 'crowding')

Dentists classify malocclusions into three broad categories, depending on the relative positions of the upper and lower jaws in relation to each other while in biting position. One or more of the above-mentioned forms of misalignment accompanies each of these following jaw positions:

Class I: Where the opposing molar teeth meet each other normally.

Class II: Where the lower jaw is recessed vis-à-vis the upper jaw, causing the chin to be drawn back.

Class III: Where the lower jaw protrudes beyond the upper

jaw, causing the chin to jut out, and the lower front teeth get into a cross bite.

If there is a major discrepancy in the relative shape or size of the upper or lower jaws, the teeth may be in serious malocclusion. This is known as a skeletal malocclusion, and surgery will be required to realign the jaws.

Problems Associated with Misaligned Teeth: Under Pressure

When teeth are not in fitting order, they can cause several problems:

- They look disagreeable, and lead to personality issues like low self-esteem.
- Chewing firm foods may become difficult.
- Some teeth can suffer excessive wear and tear.
- Crowded teeth create issues in maintaining oral hygiene.
- Protruding teeth are more prone to chipping and injury.
- Open bites cause speech defects, such as lisping.
- Gum problems can develop, such as gum recession or pockets.
- Increased incidences of dental caries occur due to improper contact between adjacent teeth.
- Incorrect biting positions can stress the joint of the jaws (the temporomandibular joint), leading to pain and increased muscle tension.

The term 'orthodontic' literally means 'straight teeth'! Orthodontic treatment basically involves the application of gentle, sustained pressure on the teeth, to move them into more desirable positions.

Broadly, this can be accomplished by the use of certain removable devices that press on the teeth, or by fixing wires and elastic bands onto them to guide them into their newly appointed places. Such pressure is transferred to the jawbone, which accommodates and changes shape by yielding to it. This results in a gradual, safe shifting of the teeth into new settings.

While most dentists can handle minor corrections, the majority of cases are best left to specialists known as orthodontists.

The Ideal Time for Orthodontic Treatment: Age No Bar

Orthodontic treatment can be done at any age! Most people assume that it is only for kids. While it is true that it can be done most effectively and efficiently in the preteen/teenage range, there is really no age restriction. It is just that tooth movements in adults can take more time, as the jawbone is denser. Also, since all the teeth would already be in place, some could require removal to create space for corrections. Adults could also shy away from orthodontic treatment, due to embarrassment amongst their peers for wearing braces.

Fortunately, modern orthodontic options include cosmetic braces, as well as those placed on the inner aspects of the teeth (lingual orthodontics) and near-invisible devices, to align them. As a result, an increasing number of adults are now undergoing orthodontic treatment, if they have missed the bus in childhood!

The ideal time, of course, is between the ages of seven and twelve, while the permanent teeth are erupting, and any apparent malocclusion can be nipped in the bud. Coupled with this, is the immense advantage of the overall evolvement of the body that takes place at this stage. The orthodontist can plan the sequence of the procedures based on these periods of development, known as growth spurts. This often helps avoid extraction of permanent teeth that might otherwise have become necessary in creating space for realignment.

Interceptive Orthodontics: Nipping It in the Bud

If any malocclusion is detected, therapy can be implemented in phases, creating favourable conditions for better alignment. This is known as 'interceptive orthodontics', and the results of such a therapy are far more impressive than those of corrective therapy alone.

Several existing and emerging problems can be attended to, in the early phases of interceptive therapy:

- Habits like thumb-sucking, if persistent, causes protrusion of the upper front teeth, along with the underlying jawbone. This may need to be remedied with the use of an orthodontic device, known as a 'habit-breaking appliance'. Similarly, habits like tongue thrusting, lip biting, mouth breathing, etc. can also be addressed.
- In some children, the upper palate is narrow, and this could lead to a cross bite, where the lower teeth overlap the upper. Early orthodontic treatment, known as palatal expansion to widen the narrow palate, prevents this from developing into a serious malocclusion later.
- If crowding of teeth is detected, orthodontic therapy will expand the size of the jaw to accommodate the teeth, so that unnecessary tooth removal is avoided in future.
- Problems like missing permanent teeth, or extra (supernumerary) teeth can prevent the development of a good alignment. Similarly, some permanent teeth,

such as the canines, can get embedded at an odd angle inside the jawbone. It is possible to address these conditions with appropriate treatments.

- If any of the milk teeth are overstaying, removing them will make way for the permanent ones waiting to erupt.
- Some children require premature removal of their milk molars due to extensive decay. Orthodontists fit a device known as a 'space maintainer' to preserve the vacated space for the succeeding permanent tooth to erupt into.
- When orthodontists diagnose an emerging malocclusion, they can formulate a time-plan for the removal of selected milk teeth, to coincide with and facilitate the natural erupting arrangements of permanent ones. This is known as 'serial extraction'.

This early phase of therapy is followed by an interim resting period, till all the permanent teeth erupt, usually by age the of twelve. During this interval, the orthodontist keeps an eye on the developing tooth alignment and growth of the jaws.

In the second phase, comprehensive orthodontic therapy can be staged when all the permanent teeth have come out (around the age of twelve). This phase can be completed quickly and efficiently, due to the interventions during the early phase.

The Duration of Orthodontic Treatment: Falling in Line Takes Time

Orthodontic treatment uses the principle of gentle pressure applied to the teeth, over extended periods of time. This allows teeth to move safely and predictably through the jawbone.

Once they reach their planned positions, they need to be held there till they settle in fully. This line of treatment, therefore, takes time to produce the desired results.

The actual period for completion depends on several factors. Here are some of the main ones:

The Age at Which Treatment Is Initiated

Naturally, the process is faster in kids, as the bone is more pliable, and the general growth phases can be utilized to guide the teeth efficiently into place. Treatment for adults is more time-consuming, as tooth movements are much slower, and may involve select teeth to be extracted.

The Severity of the Malocclusion

Needless to say, simpler corrections can be done quickly, while severe maladjustments could take much longer.

Whether There Is a Skeletal Component to the Malocclusion

If the issue occurs solely on account of the position of the teeth, rectification is swifter, but if there is a problem regarding jaw size or shape, it would involve a much longer period.

Oral Hygiene Maintenance During Treatment

Plaque and tartar accumulating on the teeth can lead to gum inflammation and bleeding. This interferes with orthodontic treatment procedures, leading to delay.

Compliance with All Instructions Related to the Treatment

Orthodontic treatment needs the full cooperation of the patient! It is a joint effort with the doctor, and if the directions are not adhered to, it will invariably end in a time lag.

This procedure can take anywhere between fifteen to

twenty-eight months, based on the factors outlined above. However, on an average, one can be prepared for a duration of around two years. Most cases that overshoot the original estimated time can be attributed to poor compliance with the orthodontist's orders (understandably the case with preteens and teens).

Devices Used for Orthodontic Treatment: Brace Yourself!

The first visit to an orthodontist is recommended by the age of seven. This helps catch problems early, and institute remedial measures at the opportune time. But, even if you miss this time slot, it is never too late to start!

The first step during the initial assessment is a thorough examination of the teeth, mouth and jaws. If the orthodontist concludes that treatment is necessary, impressions of the teeth are taken, to make plaster models for analysis. X-rays of the teeth, jaws and the entire skull help him to study various parameters. Photographs of the existing condition of the teeth, the facial contours and the profile are filed away for future comparisons.

The treatment is planned based on the analysis of these records, which dictate the course of action. Several options are available, in terms of orthodontic devices, or appliances.

Removable Appliances

These are simple orthodontic devices that are capable of addressing minor misalignments of the teeth, but incapable of precise tooth movements. They usually comprise an acrylic plate, onto which wires or springs are attached, and which is easily removed for cleaning.

These are commonly used when the milk teeth are

present, or while the permanent teeth are erupting; they can be used for adults too. Requiring to be worn for several hours daily, the desired modifications are achieved anywhere from six to nine months of use.

A recent addition to this category is a system of 'clear tooth aligners', which also achieve minor amendments such as relieving mild crowding or spacing worries. Custom-designed using computerized protocols, it consists of a sequence of clear plastic aligners called trays, which are fitted to the teeth to induce slight movements in them. Each of these needs to be worn for several hours a day, for about two to three weeks, and induces a minor tooth realignment. This is followed by the next tray, which accomplishes the next round of re-ordering, and so on. The results may be seen from between three weeks to six months, depending on the degree of change required.

Aligners are virtually invisible, and have the convenience of being removable, which facilitates cleaning. They also cause no irritation to the gums, and allow users to brush and floss their teeth normally.

Fixed Braces

These are the mainstay of orthodontic treatment, used extensively for ameliorating malocclusions. Fixed braces use a variety of elements to achieve the desired tooth movements

Archwire

A pre-shaped wire of pre-determined shape and tension is fixed to the teeth to induce the planned shifts. Initially, a flexible version is applied, to effect a

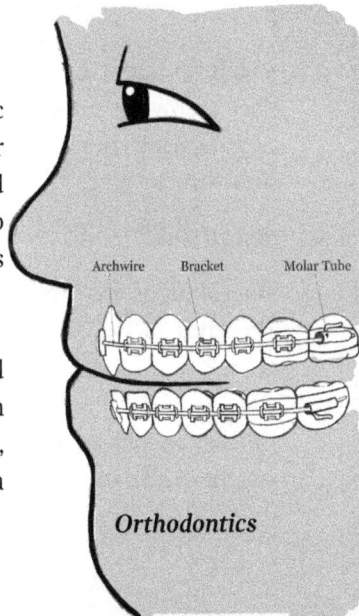

Archwire   Bracket   Molar Tube

Orthodontics

gentle realignment, following which stiffer wires are employed to exert precise controls over teeth positions. Archwires could be metallic (stainless steel or nickel-titanium) or cosmetic (metallic with tooth-coloured coatings, or non-metallic fibre reinforced polymers).

Orthodontic Bracket

This is a mooring for the archwire. Metallic, clear or tooth-coloured, it is fixed to each tooth with strong adhesive, and the archwire courses through them. (Previously, individual teeth were wrapped with a steel band, to which the bracket was anchored!)

Band

Some teeth, normally molars, may still need to be wrapped with a band, which could be of stainless steel or tooth-coloured material. They are fixed to the teeth with dental adhesive cements.

Ligature

Ligatures are tiny wires or elastic rubber bands that hold the archwire securely within the brackets (some newer 'self-ligating' brackets have an inbuilt design for keeping the archwire in place).

Buccal Tube

Buccal tubes are thin pipes fixed to bands on molars, to which the ends of the archwire are firmly detained.

Spring

Springs are placed between brackets to exert a sideways pressure on the teeth, in order to open or close spaces between them.

Elastic

Elastics are rubber bands that are run between hooks attached to the brackets of the upper and lower teeth, in order to move them into the correct chewing alignment.

Headgear

Here is a device that fits around the head or neck, and can be connected to another section that is fixed inside the mouth. This is useful in pulling the upper molars further back, to relieve crowded teeth and to correct discrepancies in jaw alignment.

Mini Implant

Mini implants have gained acceptance for orthodontic use in recent times, and are used as fixed points from which force can be applied to shift teeth. Known as 'temporary anchorage devices', they are removed after the orthodontic course is over.

The Orthodontic Session: The Belt and Braces Approach

Fixing the braces onto the teeth is usually completed in one session. Here is a typical sequence:

- The teeth are first cleaned and polished.
- They are then dried, and isolated with a plastic cheek retractor, to keep the lips and cheeks away from them.
- The tooth surface is chemically roughened or etched, using an acid.
- The brackets are then bonded onto the etched surface of each tooth with a dental adhesive.
- Finally, the archwire is strung through the brackets, and fixed in place with the ligatures. The ends of the

archwire are inserted into the molar tubes and locked in. That's it!

The orthodontist will advise a patient regarding the next visit, which is usually after four to six weeks. At every follow-up, he/she evaluates the progress, and makes adjustments to the braces initiating the next sequence of tooth movements.

Post-Orthodontic Treatment Care: Please Get This Straight Too

Mild pain in the teeth is common when braces are first applied, or after follow-up sessions when they are tightened. The insides of the lips and cheeks may also feel sore due to their contact with the brackets and wires. Mild painkillers help ease this initial pain, while a blob of orthodontic wax coating the braces, relieves the soreness. Temporary inconveniences, they settle down in a few days.

The dentist or orthodontist will provide a detailed list of strict instructions to be followed, so that the treatment progresses as planned. The most important instructions follow:

- Maintain excellent oral hygiene around the braces. After getting braces, routine cleansing gets complicated, and extra effort is required. Special orthodontic toothbrushes are available to help clean around the braces, and threaders to run floss under the archwires. In addition, small interdental brushes may be helpful to clean under the wires, while water jets or oral irrigators, are employed in removing debris from the fixed appliances.
- Use the elastics or headgear as and when applicable, and wear the removable appliances for the specified

number of hours every day. If the appliance contains a screw module for expanding the jaw, the orthodontist will advise the patient on the manner and the required intervals, for turning the screw.

- Immediately report any breakage or dislodging of any part of the braces, as it can stall the treatment and will need to be fixed right away.
- Sticky foods can dislodge the braces, and interrupt treatment. Typically, caramel-based toffees, chewy bars, pizza, etc. are best avoided.
- Hard foods can break the brackets or other components of the fixed braces. Nuts, firm fruit like apples, chunky or crunchy foods, etc. should be eaten in small cut sections to prevent such damage. Biting on ice is a strict no-no, as chewing on pencils!
- Sugary foods should be restricted, as the braces can predispose the teeth to cavity formation. Sweetened aerated beverages are particularly harmful, and should be avoided.

Removable Retainers: Work in Progress

At the end of the treatment, the teeth would have assumed their final designated positions, and the jaws would have achieved a perfect harmonious relationship with each other. The braces are then removed, and the teeth cleaned thoroughly to eliminate the bonding residues. Everything's looking good, but the treatment's not over yet!

Just as you're getting ready to party, the orthodontist takes impressions of your teeth once again, this time to fabricate retainers. These are removable appliances generally, which hold the teeth in their new places, preventing the reversal or relapse of the entire exercise. The teeth are allowed to settle in and acclimatize themselves to the forces unique to their current locations.

Removable retainers constitute an acrylic plate, with attached wires and clamps that hold on to the teeth, keeping them in position. They can cause an alteration of speech, as well as increased salivation—temporary issues, which resolve automatically in a few days. Some retainers are also made of vacuum-formed rigid plastics that fit over all the teeth.

Fixed retainers are in the form of wires which are bonded to the inside surfaces of the upper and lower front teeth. They are more convenient than removable ones, but need extra attention to clean around them.

Generally, removable retainers are used for at least a year after completion of treatment. Fixed retainers need to be left in place for about five years.

Orthodontics and Surgical Intervention: Going under the Knife

Sometimes, surgical intervention may be required to complement orthodontic treatment. This commonly involves removal of impacted teeth, exposing buried teeth or correcting gum-related problems.

Occasionally, there is serious discrepancy in the size and shape of the jaws in relation to each other, leading to misalignments, not amenable to orthodontic remedy alone. Orthognathic surgery, for jaw corrections, is required in such cases. This is usually preceded by orthodontic treatment to get the teeth into favourable positions. Post the surgery, a second phase of orthodontics follows to align the teeth into their final and desired positions.

Orthodontic Treatment, Drawbacks and Complications: Getting Your Wires Crossed

As with any form of treatment, there could be drawbacks and complications with orthodontic procedures too. Some of the major concerns are:

Unsightly Appearance

A mouth full of metal and wires doesn't lend itself to a pleasant appearance. Recent advances with clear and tooth-coloured braces are an attempt to overcome the 'metal mouth' epithet.

Long Duration of Treatment

By its very nature, orthodontic treatment is a protracted procedure, as teeth must be moved gently and gradually. This prolonged therapy can be fairly tedious, as it calls for enhanced compliance and discipline over extended periods.

High Cost

Because orthodontic treatment is a lengthy process, requiring special training, equipment, materials and expertise to ensure good results, it is expensive. Normally this load is not borne by insurance either, and can strain personal finances. However, most orthodontists offer options for paying in instalments all through the treatment period

Associated Dental Disease

The presence of braces challenges oral hygiene procedures. Usually, this means inadequate attention to cleaning the teeth, and leads to gum disease. Similarly, if not cleaned well after meals, braces allow food and sugary residues to remain in contact with the teeth for long intervals, promoting cavity formation. This can range from superficial chalky-white discolouration of the teeth to deep decay.

Incorrect Technique

If the treatment is not executed with the requisite skill and care, it can damage the teeth. Excessive force can cause them to shake, or to shorten their roots. On rare occasions, the dental pulp may die out, rendering the tooth 'non-vital'.

Modern orthodontics contributes immensely to a pleasing countenance, by improving the facial structure. In a safe, predictable manner, it also aids the ease of chewing, vital for good nutrition and health, through correct alignment of the teeth and jaws. The results are life long, and can dramatically heighten self-confidence. So, even in today's wireless world, it's time to get wired!

Chapter 18

Aesthetics in Dentistry: Glowing with Health

A 1,000-watt smile can set a room on fire! You would've certainly met people whose faces get transformed when they smile.

There's no escaping the fact that in today's world, appearance does matter! Your smile can multiply your face value many times over. The way you feel about your smile contributes immensely to your happiness quotient. Sometimes, minor imperfections can still look charming, and healthy well-aligned teeth manage to pass muster even if they are yellowish in colour.

But, there are many amongst us whose self-esteem and confidence are shot to the ground, as they try to hide their crooked, discoloured, or missing teeth.

Fortunately, it is possible to get their teeth back to looking as nature intended them to. Most procedures in dentistry strive to restore teeth to a state of good health, and to accomplish this with a strong dose of aesthetics!

Cosmetic Therapy: Look Good, Feel Good

Broadly speaking, apart from the more functional dental treatments for pain and discomfort, all others could easily fall into the category of cosmetic therapy! In recent times, a new specialty known as cosmetic dentistry has taken the placid dental world by storm! Thanks to this, perfect smiles leap out at you from the covers of glossies, white teeth dazzle you with their brilliance, and almost make you wonder why *you* don't have that striking smile.

Before we explore the niche domain of cosmetic dentistry, let's first look at the different forms of dental treatment that can produce agreeable results as well. Several procedures, in the course of restoring function, also help in lifting the smile, and thereby the overall charm. For example, getting an inexpensive removable denture for a front tooth that got knocked out can be highly cosmetic!

Cosmetic Therapy, Tooth Extraction and Oral Surgery: Stranger than Fiction

Strange as it may sound, a tooth extraction, on occasion, may render a cosmetic benefit! There could be an extra front tooth, known as a mesiodens, which sits bang between the two front incisors. Removing this can dramatically boost one's appearance.

Tooth extractions also pave the way for the next line of treatment. Damaged or mutilated teeth in the visible zone need to be removed, before an implant or bridge, with a perfect artificial tooth, can be installed. Similarly, some extractions could be required for orthodontic realignment.

A serious mismatch in the jaw sizes and alignment may beg orthognathic surgery, which can dramatically transform the face structure most positively.

Cosmetic Therapy and Orthodontics: Down to the Wire

Before the advent of cosmetic dentistry, the field of orthodontics was the uncrowned king when it came to procedures for augmenting the facial appearance! Orthodontic treatment, as we know, brings about the movement of teeth and the underlying jawbone into better functional and refined arrangements.

The cosmetic benefits of orthodontics, as we know, are diverse—crooked teeth are realigned and straightened to accord an even arrangement; the gaps between teeth are closed; and the facial shape and jawline are improved by readjusting their positioning.

These cosmetic changes are usually permanent, with little or no invasive alterations extended to the natural teeth. The flip side is that one needs to wear braces and maintain them for a rather long duration, usually around two years.

Cosmetic Therapy and Gum Treatment: In the Pink

Treatment for gum problems focuses primarily on returning them to health.

Healthy gums, perfectly posited, are a prime component of a vibrant smile! Here are some gum treatments that can help improve the appearance of gums that fail to match up.

Scaling and Polishing

This simple, routine procedure eliminates tartar deposits on the teeth, together with the dental plaque they shelter. It expels inflammation of the gums—the redness and bleeding disappear and the swelling subsides. Simultaneously, the teeth look healthier and brighter, as scaling also rids them of unsightly stains!

Gingivectomy

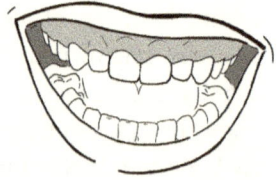

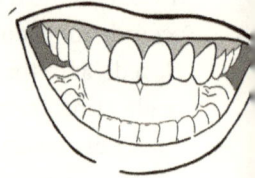

Gingivectomy

When the gum tissue has grown over and on to the teeth, it leads to a 'gummy' smile, making the teeth look short and unappealing. Such gums can be cut back under the effect of local anaesthesia, and returned to their normal state. A minor version of this procedure is called gingivoplasty, where the gums are subtly sculpted and contoured to the desired shape.

Depigmentation

Most people want pink gums! While they may be predominantly pink in colour, they can often be dark, due to melanin pigments (which are also responsible for the colour of our skin). Sometimes, there is excessive melanin deposition or uneven splotches, which may be of concern from an aesthetic standpoint.

A gum specialist, the periodontist, can correct this by removing the dark layer surgically, or by using lasers. The gums are restored to a preferred pink shade, but over time, there may be some recurrence.

Crown Lengthening

Occasionally, a too-short tooth may require not only the cutback of excess gum tissue, but following that, the trimming of a bit of the bone underneath it as well. To do this, the gums are peeled back to access the jawbone. The entire procedure, known as crown lengthening, is also done when a tooth needing to be crowned doesn't have the required length for the cap to get a hold on.

After a healing period of about four to six weeks, a significant increase is obtained in the visible length of the tooth.

Frenectomy

Some front teeth have wide spaces between them, which look unseemly. At times, this is due to the pull of a thin fold of inner lip tissue known as a frenum, which encroaches this space. Before any other corrective treatment is meted out to close the space, this tissue needs to be snipped through a minor surgery known as a frenectomy.

Gum Grafts

Sometimes, there is a significant facial drawback due to receded gums in the front teeth—they look longer and their yellower roots are exposed. Periodontists cover these receded areas with gum grafts—portions of gum tissue taken from other parts of the mouth. A similar procedure can be adopted to build up deficient gum tissue before bridging a missing tooth, eliminating the ugly gap under the artificial one!

Cosmetic Therapy and Restoration: The Rot Sets In

Dental caries looks bad! It leaves yellow, brown or black marks on teeth, and progresses to eat away the tooth structure. The result can be large black holes, which look particularly awful where the front teeth are concerned.

Treatments for these conditions include the following:
- One can opt for tooth-coloured fillings that restore teeth to their natural glory! The decay is drilled away, and the deficit filled up layer by layer, till the tooth looks

as good as the original!

- Crowns can be made to cover teeth that have lost too much structure and look mutilated. Sculpted to perfectly blend with the other teeth, these crowns are made of tooth-coloured materials—porcelain fused to metal, porcelain fused to zirconia or all-ceramic.
- Inlays and onlays are other types of tooth-coloured restorations that are devised from composite resins or porcelain, and bonded to the tooth.

Cosmetic Therapy and Tooth Replacement: No Skin off Our Teeth

Replacement of a missing tooth, especially in the front row, bestows excellent results from a cosmetic angle. In the form of dental implants, fixed bridges, or even removable dentures, all these variants can be fashioned to look absolutely lifelike, and undetectable in the normal course.

A complete denture lends a huge helping hand as far as appearance is concerned. Apart from providing teeth where none exist, it supports the sagging facial tissues, reviving the shape of the face.

In some people, severe erosion of their grinders' chewing surfaces causes the jaw to over-close. Called 'loss of vertical dimension', it causes the face look shorter, and wrinkles to appear at the corners of the mouth. This condition needs extensive rehabilitation of the teeth, with multiple crowns or bridges to raise the biting platform. The outcome—the return of the normal length of face, and disappearance of the wrinkles!

Dentists strive to bring your teeth back to health—it is their top priority. At the same time, routine dental procedures focus on maintaining your normal looks, or even in elevating them. Our next chapter on cosmetic dentistry explores this exciting world of make-believe!

CHAPTER 19

Cosmetic Dentistry:
Beauty Lies...

Ever wondered how film and television stars have those perfect teeth? Their dazzle catches your attention, and the entire smile looks oh-so perfectly proportioned. Given their chaotic schedules, you wonder how they manage to maintain those glittering pearlies.

Welcome to the world of cosmetic dentistry—the art of making teeth look beautiful! The field of cosmetic dentistry places an emphasis on procedures that focus on cultivating the appearance of the teeth—especially the visible ones—and the smile, and not on relieving pain or restoring function. This skill is still not considered a specialty by many dental professional bodies, including the American Dental Association. Thus, it comes under the purview of the general dentist.

Any skilled and experienced dental practitioner can carry out a number of cosmetic procedures, and design not just a smile, but perk up the overall confidence and self-esteem of the patient too. There are plenty who claim to be Cosmetic Dentists, and many of you will also be familiar with the term 'smile designing'—a catchword in cosmetic dentistry.

Relying strongly on the ability to create an illusion of perfection and health, broadly, three types of procedures are employed in this field:

- Colour change: This is where the inherent colour of the teeth is modified, making them lighter or whiter. Tooth whitening or bleaching procedures fall into this category.
- Subtraction: This is where teeth are subtly reshaped to create a more pleasing appearance.
- Addition: This is where tooth-coloured materials are fixed or bonded onto the teeth to change their shape, fill gaps, etc. All bonding procedures and laminates would fall into this category.

Colour Change for Teeth: Whiter than White

Yes, we know. Who doesn't want a Cindy Crawford smile—teeth dazzling like fresh snow? Today, cosmetic dentistry can offer just that. But before we get to the 'hows', let's consider the 'whys'.

Factors Influencing Tooth Colour

Did you know that everyone's teeth are a different colour? We assume that all teeth are white, but there are huge variations in the inherent hues of our teeth. In fact, there are perhaps more shades in teeth as compared to human skin! Many factors influence the colour of our teeth, some genetic, some acquired:

Race

Fair-skinned people tend to have yellower teeth than dark-skinned folk. Some studies have attributed the relative contrast between skin and tooth colour as the reason for this 'perception'.

Age

Milk teeth are very white! Is it any surprise, then, that they are called milk teeth? The difference between them and permanent teeth can be seen most tellingly in children, when the latter start replacing the milk teeth. The contrast is quite remarkable, with the whiter milk teeth, juxtaposed to the 'yellower' permanent ones! Hence, parents often complain that their child is not brushing their teeth well enough.

Permanent teeth are lighter when they arrive, as their thick covering layer of enamel reflects light. As we grow older, there is gradual thinning of the enamel due to routine wear and tear. This brings the inner layer, the dentin, closer to the surface. Dentin is yellower than enamel, and absorbs light, making it look darker. Over the years, micro-cracks can appear in the teeth, giving them an aged, weathered look.

Habits

We subject our teeth to many stain-causing substances, such as coffee, dark fruit juices and red wine. Other culprits include habits like smoking, or chewing tobacco, betel nut and pan masala.

Internal Stains

Teeth, in which the dental pulp dies out due to infection or injury, can get stained internally. The breakdown of haemoglobin in the blood vessels of such teeth causes the brown pigments to leach into the tooth. Certain medications (for instance, tetracycline) taken in childhood, while the teeth are only just forming, can also lead to internal discolouration. If you were exposed, again as a child, to very high levels of fluoride in drinking water, you could have developed dental fluorosis, causing staining and pitting of teeth.

Teeth Whitening Procedures

A recipe for tooth whitening: Take a spoonful of ground pumice. Mix well with half an ounce of wine vinegar to make a thick paste. Rub this paste on your teeth with your forefinger, and sit in the shade of a pyramid. Yes, you guessed right—this recipe is about 5,000 years old from ancient Egypt, and is not recommended unless you have a pyramid at hand!

Humans seem to have been dissatisfied with the colour of their teeth from time immemorial. Even the Romans, it is believed, used urine to whiten their teeth (the active ingredient being ammonia). For obvious reasons, this therapy is also not strongly recommended.

So, what's the best way to get those dazzlers, and safely? Some techniques include:

- A tooth whitening procedure performed at the dental clinic, known as 'in-office bleach'
- A process which starts at the dental clinic, but whose active phase you accomplish at home, called 'dentist-supervised home bleach'
- A dental procedure for non-vital or dead teeth
- A range of miscellaneous over-the-counter options and dental procedures

Before the teeth are taken up for any whitening procedures, the dentist will do a complete examination of the mouth. It is important to first figure out the reason for the dark colour of the teeth, and whether the discolouration will respond to bleaching procedures. Some conditions may have to be treated differently.

The dentist will also check for the presence of restorations, crowns, etc. If they are leaky, they must be corrected to prevent discomfort during the bleaching process. Any prevailing tooth sensitivity is kept in mind, as the bleach programme should be modified to minimize pain in such instances. Besides, cavities, if any, must be appropriately restored, prior to tooth whitening procedures.

The dentist records the existing shade of the teeth, so that the final results can be compared. Once all this is done and dusted, a thorough scaling and polishing process is carried out to eliminate superficial stains, and to get the gums into a state of health.

In-office Bleach

This procedure is discharged at the dental clinic, and is a quick fix with rapid results. Usually, the treatment is restricted to the eight to ten visible teeth—up to the premolars. The dentist uses high-concentration bleaches, the commonest formulation being a hydrogen peroxide gel, at around 35 per cent concentration.

First, the gums are protected with a covering barrier material, as the bleach can cause them chemical burns. The bleaching gel is then placed on the tooth/teeth, and left in place for fifteen to twenty minutes.

Some operators believe that activating the gel through exposure to a strong light source enhances the bleaching effect, for which halogen, LED lights and lasers are the various options exercised.

The gel is washed off after the first cycle, and a second similar cycle is initiated. Most operators prefer a total sitting of one hour, spanning three application cycles. At the end of this, a radical improvement in the colour of the teeth is realized—lightened by three to eight shades!

This is obviously the preferred choice for people pressed for time, as the results are effective and quick. Specific teeth that need extra whitening can also be managed better, since it is under the control of the dentist.

The negatives are that the teeth could become sensitive, as high power chemicals are used, and if the protective barrier on the gums is not placed carefully enough, they will suffer serious chemical injury. Also, for those desirous of greater improvement, repeat sessions may need to be scheduled.

Dentist-supervised Home Bleach

This is a gentler, slower procedure for whitening your teeth, and can be done entirely at your own convenience! The dentist's and the patient's roles are clearly demarcated.

• The Dentist's Role
The dentist first takes impressions of your teeth to make a replica known as a model or cast. Using this model, a vinyl mould—called a bleaching tray—is fabricated, which is like a transparent jacket that closely fits your teeth. The dentist checks the fit of this tray on your teeth, and adjustments are made, as necessary, to ensure that it is favourable.
The dentist provides the bleaching gel kit: the gel packaged in user-friendly syringes, and the nozzles for fixing on to them. The gels generally comprise 10 to 22 per cent carbamide peroxide, which translates into a 3.5 to 7 per cent concentration of hydrogen peroxide.
The dentist demonstrates to you the technique for applying the bleaching gel into the tray, with the syringe and nozzle present in the kit. Typically, dentists recommend bleaching either the upper or lower teeth one at a time, as it can get uncomfortable holding two bleaching trays together in the

mouth. Also, this way you can gauge the whitening effect by comparing the bleached teeth with the unbleached.

• Your Role at Home
  Follow the instructions, and inject the gel into the bleaching tray. Place the tray into the correct position on your teeth, as demonstrated by your dentist. The excess gel that leaches out onto the gums needs to be immediately cleaned out with cotton gauze, to prevent irritation.
  The tray can be worn overnight, or for a couple of hours during the day, after which, it is to be removed, thoroughly cleaned, and kept aside till the next use.
  Results are obtained after several sessions, over one to four weeks, depending on the strength of the gel.
  The effects of this process are predictable, and highly effective. Missed sessions, which do not impact the final results—can be covered up later. And, since it uses milder gels, tooth sensitivity is less of an issue too.
  The drawback is the time factor, due to the need for repeated applications. Also, specific teeth, which may need extra attention, cannot be catered to, as the effect is more generalized.

Here are some of the instructions you need to follow for the home-bleach process.

The dos:

• Always brush and floss your teeth before bleaching them to remove plaque, as clean tooth surfaces ensure better penetration of the bleaching gel into the enamel.
• After the prescribed time, remove the bleaching tray from the mouth, and do clean your teeth as usual.
• The bleaching tray must be cleaned before and after use.

- You could use desensitizing mouthwashes or toothpastes for a few days, till the related sensitivity abates. Rarely, analgesics will be prescribed if the pain is severe.

The don'ts:

- Avoid drinking water with the bleach tray in the mouth.
- Stay away from foods that stain the teeth, like colas, tea, coffee, red wine, etc.
- Quit smoking and other forms of tobacco use.
- Stop chewing paan, betel nut or paan masala.
- During and immediately after the bleaching procedure, avoid food items and beverages at extremes of temperature, as the teeth will be sensitive. In case this problem of tooth-sensitivity persists, the dentist may prescribe desensitizing gels to be included in the bleaching trays.

Whitening for Non-vital or Dead Teeth

When the pulp dies out in a tooth, it could leave behind grave discolouration from the ensuing blood debris. Before attending to this issue, such teeth need to first receive a root canal treatment.

After this is done, the dentist will, in a procedure known as 'walking bleach', remove a part of the root filling, replace it with the bleaching agent, and seal it. The bleach is allowed to work its magic over a few days. Two or more repeat applications may be necessary at seven to ten day intervals. Once the desired lightening has taken place, the bleach material is removed, a permanent filling material replaced, and the cavity once again sealed.

The discoloured tooth can also be tackled by a regular in-office procedure, by applying a concentrated bleach gel on it.

A combination technique can be used, where the tooth is opened up as in the 'walking bleach' technique, and the bleach chemicals applied both inside and outside to whiten the tooth inside out.

Other Teeth Whitening Procedures

The whitening procedures we have listed can yield good results, and eliminate the need for hiding the discolouration with crowns or veneers, bringing down the cost of treatment. However, serious discolourations may not respond, and other options would have to be explored.

Whitening of teeth is not a one-time procedure! It may need to be repeated after a few years, as teeth tend to discolour again over time. Some dentists perform an in-office bleach, and then recommend continuing with a home-bleach programme for more sustained results.

In a dental set up, the dentist proffers a crucial value-addition by studying the teeth, and their suitability for whitening procedures. Your fillings and crowns are checked to ensure their integrity. Tooth sensitivity, can be quickly addressed, else it would which may be troublesome during the bleach process.

With do-it-yourself programmes, you are basically on your own. A variety of over-the-counter bleach preparations are available which employ the same chemicals used in professional situations, but need to be used with caution. Often, they end up in inadequate whitening, irritation and injury to the gums, and sensitive teeth. Some of these formulations are similar to the home-bleach options, but come with non-customized bleach trays, which don't fit accurately, compromising the results, and causing gum irritation.

Plastic bleach-coated whitening strips are also available.

These need to be placed on the teeth for about thirty minutes a day, to release the bleach chemicals into them. But the strips tend to fall off, and the saliva weakens the bleach action. Gum irritation is also common.

An array of whitening toothpastes is found in the market. These usually combine abrasives with bleach chemicals, but since they don't remain in contact with the teeth for long, the results are not sustained.

Tooth Recontouring: Whipping Things into Shape

This is another technique used in cosmetic dentistry to enhance the appearance of teeth. The procedure is known as enameloplasty or odontoplasty wherein small amounts of tooth enamel are selectively removed to deliver the desired effect. This is a slightly more invasive technique for designing one's smile, as opposed to bleaching, which is virtually non-invasive.

Tooth recontouring is implemented in the following situations:

- When there is a small chip or break in a front tooth, it can be gently leveled off.
- If one tooth is longer than the rest, it can be brought in line with the others.
- Canines that are too sharp or too long can make you look predatory! Recontouring their points delivers a more human look.
- If the surface of a tooth has any bulges or pits, these can be smoothed down to normalize its appearance.
- When adjacent teeth are crowded up, they can be made to look more orderly, by gentle reshaping of their side surfaces.

Dentists use fine tools like sanding disks or diamond polishing burs, to delicately trim away the enamel. Care is taken to remove only the enamel, and to not expose the dentin, which can make the tooth sensitive.

Recontouring produces immediate results! It is fast, and doesn't cause any tooth sensitivity. The drawback is that it has limited applications, and can only be used for subtle corrections.

Bonding: Spit and Polish

This refers to the process of permanently affixing materials matching with the shade of the tooth, to either change its appearance or to fill a cavity. The most commonly used substance is the composite resin, which we discussed in the section on fillings in Chapter Twelve.

Composite resins are truly wonderful materials—they are highly polishable, developing a glossy sheen and come in an array of shades, ensuring a perfect match for almost any natural tooth colour! Dentists love it: they can place it on the tooth, sculpt, mould and smoothen it to the desired shape, and harden it in a jiffy by flashing a light on it.

While it adds grace to fillings in decayed teeth, bonding can be done for healthy teeth too, to enhance their appearance. Its versatile nature allows it to be applied in numerous situations:

- Chipped or fractured teeth can be repaired.
- Misaligned teeth can be made to look straighter, without actually straightening them.
- The shape of teeth can be changed.
- Malformed teeth can be given a normal look.
- The length of short or worn-down teeth can be increased.

- Gaps between teeth can be closed.
- Discoloured teeth, which may not respond to bleach procedures, can be bonded over.

Bonding is a chair-side procedure—basically, the dentist completes the task there and then in the clinic, without needing to refer any processing to a dental laboratory. Even when extensive changes are planned, the dentist can make models of your teeth after taking their impressions; the proposed work can be simulated on these, with the dentist and you, together, planning your designer smile.

Before bonding, the tooth surface is cleaned well to remove all depositions. Some procedures can be executed without any removal of existing enamel, or any anaesthetic either. In situations where the tooth surface needs to be cut back, local anaesthesia may be needed.

The bond to the teeth is achieved by using an adhesive, known as a bonding agent. After this is applied on the tooth, the composite resin is layered over it, and moulded and shaped as necessary. It is then cured (hardened) by exposure to a light-cure machine, or through lasers. The new look is created within minutes!

The bonding is then polished to acquire its healthy gloss and at the end, a sealant is painted on as the finishing touch, to protect the teeth from bacteria and stains.

Bonding has many advantages—it can be completed in a single visit, gives very good aesthetic results, and is less expensive than crowns or laminates.

There are a few demerits too—bonding can chip, fracture or discolour over time, and may need to be redone in a few years.

Porcelain Laminates: Glossing over Things

Porcelain laminates or veneers are ultra-thin shells of porcelain, which are made to fit on the front surfaces of your teeth. They are custom-fabricated in dental laboratories, and serve the same cosmetic purposes as bonding.

The procedure is different from that used for bonding. Local anaesthesia may or may not be necessary, depending on the sensitivity level of the teeth to the minimal drilling required. The front surfaces of the teeth are thinned down by about half a millimeter, to create a corresponding space for accommodating the thickness of the laminate.

Next, the dentist takes accurate impressions of the prepared teeth, and sends them along with the desired colour (called the shade) to the dental laboratory, which then prepares the laminates in a ceramic furnace. Porcelain veneers can be made in two ways, the traditional layered technique, or a newer pressed technique. Pressed ceramic veneers are stronger, better fitting and kinder to the opposing natural teeth than layered veneers, but necessitate a little more shaving of the tooth.

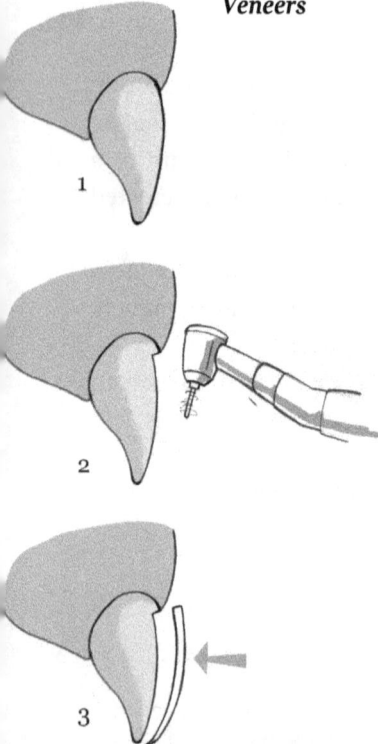

Veneers

After making any needed adjustments to the veneers, the dentist fixes them to the teeth with special adhesive cements, which create a strong bond between the two.

Porcelain veneers are the preferred choice of dentists for achieving the picture-perfect smiles we see in celebrities! Their translucency is the closest to our tooth enamel, and therefore, looks the most natural. They are also extremely durable, and don't stain or discolour as in bonding.

However, porcelain laminates are expensive! Not only that, but multiple steps are entailed in completing the process, and skilled laboratory support essential for ensuring a good finish. And *you* need to be careful—porcelain veneers can break if you bite on hard stuff. No chomping into tough nuts, ice, and bone!

A relatively new introduction is the concept of 'no-prep' veneers—they are ultra-thin (for instance, Lumineers™, Vivaneers™ and Durathin™), and can be affixed without having to pare down the teeth. Leaving the natural tooth surface intact under the veneer, these are suitable for minor corrections, as the thinness limits their versatility. Also, the teeth can feel 'thicker' after donning them.

Home Care for Cosmetic Treatment

The long-term results of cosmetic dentistry depend a lot on the home care of teeth. Daily oral care practices like brushing twice and flossing are mandatory, as is a biannual dental checkup.

As we now know, the colour of the treated teeth can be maintained by avoiding excessive intake of tea, coffee, colas, and red wine, all of which leave stains. Smoking and other forms of tobacco usage cause heavy discolouration, and compromise cosmetic interventions.

Biting into hard foods with the front teeth is best avoided, as the bonding or veneers can chip or break, or even come off entirely.

Cosmetic dental procedures have opened up several possibilities for enhancing and beautifying the teeth. At the same time, they need to be resorted to only in appropriate situations—for example, while they can improve the look of some misaligned teeth, they cannot always be a substitute for orthodontic treatment.

Since many of the cosmetic procedures, like whitening and bonding, could be want-based rather than need-based, it is important to have a clear idea of your expectations and the possible results. It is wisest to heed the advice of your dentist, so that you can get the finest smile that money can buy!

Chapter 20

Dental Checkups:
Teeth and More

Car servicing, preventive maintenance of air-conditioners, replacement of filters on water purifiers—we attend to these diligently, and even set up alarms to remind us. However, most of us miss a crucial biannual schedule—a dental review!

The Need for Regular Dental Care: Fighting Tooth and Nail

Our teeth need professional attention every six months, for several reasons:

- Cavity formation can occur at any age, and we ought to keep a lifelong vigil over this possibility. Cavities take time to form, and a six-monthly check allows early detection and treatment.
- Tartar deposits also amass over time, despite your following a good routine of oral hygiene. It allows gum disease to set in—your teeth need professional cleaning twice a year to keep that at bay!
- Good oral hygiene practices are the best way to keep your teeth healthy—your dentist can monitor your efforts during routine checkups, and help you rectify any deficiency.

- The dentist can also examine your fillings, crowns, bridges, dentures, implants, etc., to ensure that they are in good condition. If not, then further treatment will be required.
- Tooth grinding (bruxism) is a common habit, and the dentist can check for tooth wear and damage to the temporomandibular joint during your checkup.

Teeth as Mirrors of the Body: Elementary, My Dear!

Apart from the focus on teeth, gums and the jaws, dentists also

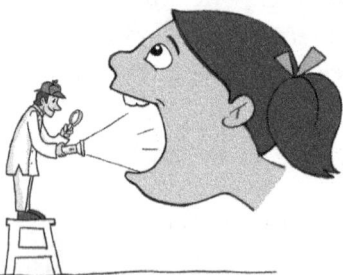

look for other signs. The mouth is the mirror of the human body. Often, the dentist can detect signs of an ailment before even you've observed any symptoms. Here are some of the conditions he/she can notice during the routine dental examination.

Oral Cancer

India has a very high incidence of mouth cancer, and most cases are detected by dentists. Ninety per cent of people who suffer from this disease have one thing in common: all of them use tobacco! Another alarming fact: for every hundred cases of oral cancer worldwide, eighty-six are from India!

Here's another amazing fact: India has a Tobacco Promotion Board, whose primary aim is to support tobacco growers, promote use of tobacco and develop new markets overseas for our indigenous produce!

Isn't it ironical then, that the government itself spends huge amounts of money on awareness campaigns against tobacco use? Short films on its ills are screened in every cinema theatre. Gory images of mouth cancer are mandatory on all tobacco products, with a statutory warning, leaving no doubt about tobacco being the leading cause of mouth cancer.

Millions of rupees are spent on government-sponsored or subsidized treatment for the disease in our country—a serious drain on the national exchequer. Why would we then have a board to protect tobacco manufacturing and marketing interests?

Factors Causing Oral Cancer

In our societies, tobacco use has found widespread acceptance through the ages. While largely consumed by adults earlier, young children are the latest victims. Thousands of poor people use tobacco as a hunger suppressant, and for this reason, it is given to their kids too. Tobacco use is now rampant, and there are many forms in which it is used. Let's consider these, as well as other factors that may make us risk-prone.

• Cigarettes, Beedis, Pipes and Hookahs
  This is one of the most underrated addictions—while there is still some social stigma associated with alcohol addiction, smoking is not constrained by any such consideration—there is simply no brouhaha when people smoke! In fact, there is a 'cool' factor associated with it, and peer pressure inducts new recruits too.
  Smoking has various avatars: cigarette, beedi, pipe, hookah, chillum and cheroot. All forms of smoking (whether filtered or non-filtered) are harmful. Apart from its carcinogenic properties, the nicotine and tar ingredients damage the delicate mouth tissues, and the heat from smoking causes smokers to develop dark lips. Smoking saps your energy,

and causes a dry mouth, which, as you now know, breeds bacteria.

Globally, thankfully, there is now a ban on smoking in public places. Tobacco products are no longer advertised, or endorsed by celebrities who serve as role models for our youth.

- Smokeless Tobacco

Tobacco is also used in various smokeless forms. For instance, burnt tobacco ground together with ash/rice/wheat husks (with or without salt) serves as a tooth powder. Mishri is a roasted tobacco powder for cleaning the teeth, and one soon gets addicted to it.

The other most common form is the quid. Tobacco leaves and lime are mixed and applied between the teeth and the lip/cheek. This pack is often left in the mouth for hours.

Tobacco is one of the ingredients in paan/betel leaf, which is chewed. A cocktail of other variants are included, all of which are detrimental to the oral tissues—lime, tobacco, betel nut and kaththa. Another additive, gulkand (sweetened rose petals) can contribute to tooth decay too.

Gutkha, popularized as a mouth freshener, is comprised of betel nut pieces, coated with a paste of tobacco powder, slaked lime, flavouring agents and other addictive ingredients. Khaini is a mixture of powdered tobacco, lime and other flavouring agents, which is placed between the lower lip and the front teeth. None of these products can be recommended!

- Alcohol

Apart from tobacco, there are other causes for oral cancer too, alcohol being one of them. Alcoholics are more prone to the disease, as alcohol is a tissue irritant. They also generally smoke, worsening their chances.

- Sharp Teeth and Ill-fitting Dentures
  Long-standing irritation from sharp teeth or ill-fitting dentures has long been debated as a cause of oral cancer.

- Virus Infection
  HPV16 (the human papilloma virus) can lead to oral cancer.

- Family History
  If there is a genetic tendency for cancer in the family, one may be more likely to develop it in the mouth.

Early Pre-cancerous Signs in the Mouth

There is a group of conditions that are classified as pre-cancerous, some of the common ones being leukoplakia, erythroplakia, and oral submucous fibrosis (OSMF). Most of these are caused by habits like gutkha and tobacco consumption.

Leukoplakia appears as a white patch inside the mouth, usually on the inner cheeks or inside the lip surfaces. Erythroplakia emerges similarly, but the patch is reddish in colour. Oral submucous fibrosis is most commonly associated with gutkha chewing. The inner cheek lining becomes stiff; there is a burning sensation in the mouth, as well as difficulty in opening it, and intolerance to spicy food. Children and young adults fall prey to its consumption, especially in rural populations and amongst the urban poor. Thankfully, sale of tobacco and gutkha near schools is banned in India since a few years.

Signs and Symptoms of Oral Cancer

If the tobacco habit is discontinued, there is a good chance for the body to reverse the damage. Conversely, if the habit continues, these precancerous conditions have the potential to turn malignant.

Unfortunately many instances of oral cancer are detected in the later stages. Occasionally, by the time that happens, it is highly advanced or has even spread to other parts of the body (called metastasis).

There are warning signs present in the mouth, but they may not be painful or debilitating enough for the sufferer to seek a dentist's advice. Men are more likely to develop oral cancer than women. However, with the increase in the number of women smoking, it might soon affect them as much. People over fifty years of age are more likely to be inflicted by oral cancer as compared to youngsters.

These are some of the symptoms to watch out for:

- Inexplicable bleeding from the mouth, not necessarily from the gums
- Sore areas in the mouth
- Persistent mouth ulcers that do not heal
- Swellings, lumps/bumps inside the mouth.
- Sudden appearance of irregular growths in the mouth
- Swollen lymph nodes under the lower jaw, or neck region
- Hairy, velvety areas on the tongue, inner cheeks or lips
- White, red or wrinkled surfaces inside the mouth
- Sudden change in the fit of dentures
- Soreness or difficulty in swallowing
- Pain while swallowing or eating.
- Numbness in the tongue, lip, cheek
- Change in the voice

Diagnosis and Treatment of Oral Cancer

There are many types of oral cancers affecting any of the soft or hard bony tissues in the mouth, but one known as 'squamous cell carcinoma' is the most common. Unfortunately, oral cancers are not easily detected in the early stages, but dentists can often see the signs during dental visits and routine examinations. They can also glean much information from your history—the questionnaire that you fill up regarding your habits, symptoms, medical conditions, etc.

The mouth examination includes a thorough check of not only the teeth and gums, but of all the other soft tissues as well: the inner side of the cheeks and lips, the tongue, the palate. Dentists look for any obvious changes, which could indicate the presence of cancer.

If anything suspicious is found, the dentist can do a quick 'brush' biopsy—a special brush is rubbed on the surface of the suspicious patch to obtain a sample, which is then tested in a laboratory. This process is performed without the need for local anaesthesia. The definitive test is a standard biopsy—in other words, a small sample of the tissue is surgically removed under local anaesthesia and sent for analysis.

Once a diagnosis of oral cancer is made, treatment must start immediately. In the earlier stages, the chances of complete recovery are better. If the condition is a pre-cancerous one, stopping the offending habit can often reverse it. If not, and as the disease progresses to more advanced stages, treatment may not be successful. Aggressive interventions like surgery, cancer-fighting medications and treatments (chemotherapy), and radiation are then necessitated at the hands of oncologists, in conjunction with the dentist.

Surgery may be restricted to removing the growth, and

even some healthy tissues around it. In severe cases, part of the jaw, or the entire jaw itself, could require to be removed, to prevent the disease from spreading. When mouth cancers advance to other parts of the body, the chances of survival are bleak.

Those whose treatment has been successful are considered to be in remission: the disease is not active, but may return. Periodical follow-ups are mandatory to detect any recurrence of the cancer.

While many people consider dentistry as elitist, the purview of the rich and the urban, it is often the poor and the rural population that needs the dentist more, when it comes to oral cancer. This is because tobacco consumption in all its forms, alcoholism, malnutrition and poor oral hygiene practices are relatively more common amongst them. Sadly, they don't have the access to adequate oral healthcare facilities for timely checkups and treatment.

As tobacco usage and alcoholism are social afflictions, it is important to create increased awareness through educative programmes in schools, colleges and local governing bodies. Further, diagnostic dental checkups should be mandated in all primary health centres in our villages.

Quite a few dentists involve themselves in serving the less-fortunate members of their communities, by holding free dental health check and treatment camps. This ensures early detection of oral cancer, and increases the awareness of the disease in areas with poor oral care facilities.

While oral cancer is one of the more life-threatening conditions, a routine dental examination can sniff out the presence of other ailments that may have gone unnoticed:

Diabetes

Correctly known as diabetes mellitus, this 'lifestyle' disease affects large segments of the population today, thanks to our modern way of life: junk food, sugary diets and lack of exercise. It is a dangerous illness, as it affects the functioning of most body systems. With high sugar levels in the blood, it pushes up cardio-vascular risk, damages the kidneys and the eyes, and affects healing. Unfortunately, it is not easily detected, as there may be no outward symptoms of this illness for a long time.

As diabetes causes changes within the mouth too, dentists are often the first healthcare professionals to detect this disease. Swollen gums, gum infections, multiple gumboils, persistent bad breath, and loose teeth are pointers. Diabetics are also prone to fungal infection of the mouth. The dentist can advise a simple blood test to diagnose the condition, and then refer the case to a physician for the necessary treatment.

Blood-related Disorders

Anaemia, or deficiency of haemoglobin in the blood, has several causes. Since some of them can be fairly grave, a quick diagnosis is important. Dentists are able to discover it because the lining of the mouth and tongue becomes relatively pale, and the tongue surface can appear smooth and shiny.

Leukaemia is actually a group of conditions, commonly known as blood cancer, in which the gums become swollen, and can bleed without any provocation. Patients may seek dental treatment at first on account of these symptoms.

Vitamin Deficiency

Vitamins are important in maintaining the integrity of

our body structures and their functioning. Several vitamin deficiencies manifest with signs in the mouth—burning sensation, smooth tongue, ulceration in the mouth and at its corners, etc. Dentists can often diagnose these problems, and recommend appropriate treatment with vitamin supplements.

Heart Disease

On occasion, heart disease may present as pain in the lower jaw. Dentists are often consulted, and if they rule out any dental causes for the pain, it may be safer to consult a physician to check for heart problems.

Mouth Dryness

This common symptom has a variety of underlying causes. It could be due to medications for blood pressure, vitamin deficiency, hormonal imbalances (for instance, menopause), autoimmune disease (for instance, Sjogren's disease), salivary gland dysfunction, depression, etc. Dryness of the mouth leads to increased cavity formation and gum disease. Dentists are well placed to diagnose the problem, and suggest appropriate treatment.

Skin Disease

Some skin conditions like lichen planus, which causes itchy patches all over the body, preview in the mouth before any disturbance is noticed on the skin. The dentist can diagnose it by its typical appearance on the mouth lining, complaints of a burning mouth and an inability to tolerate spice. Treatment can be initiated, and its appearance on the skin thwarted.

Disturbances of the Digestive System

The mouth is where the digestive system begins, and can

reflect disturbances occurring in other parts of the system. Ulcerative colitis and Crohn's disease can emerge with oral changes, acid-reflux can be detected by erosion of tooth enamel, and tummy upsets can cause bad breath and mouth ulceration.

HIV

This deadly disease often displays telltale signs in the mouth—white lesions, fungal infections and reddish tumours (called Kaposi's sarcoma). Dentists can recognize these signs and steer the affected person in the right direction for treatment.

Stress

Psychological stress is a widespread condition, and can be reasonably debilitating. Dentists can detect signs of this through accelerated wear of the teeth due to bruxism, tension in the jaw muscles, clicking sounds in the temporomandibular joint, stress-linked mouth conditions like lichen planus, etc. They can help by recommending a psychologist for counseling, or in severe cases, a psychiatrist for necessary medication.

★

A myriad other illnesses leave their marks in the mouth. Dentists are trained to recognize these symptoms, and can help sufferers by pointing out the diagnosis, and paving the way for timely treatment.

Your dental checkup can ensure not only healthy teeth and gums, it can also help you to preserve your overall health—the dentist's mirror can reflect much more than just your teeth!

Chapter 21

Dentists and Patients: Great Expectations

'One thing I like less than most things is sitting in a dentist chair'—Ogden Nash's sentiments are echoed by most! Any occasion can broadly fall under one of three categories:

- The enjoyable, which you actually look forward to
- The neutral, which doesn't excite you much, but you don't mind going through it
- The unpleasant, which you tend to avoid as far as possible

For the multitude, unfortunately, a visit to the dentist falls under the last category. Many factors add up to produce this negative sentiment, which leads to postponements, and even avoidance of timely dental care.

Fear of pain during treatment, and phobias related to the dental clinic are perhaps the foremost causes, the basis for which we explored in the very first chapter of this book.

Next in line is the perceived ability to manage without teeth—it is not life-threatening, so the reluctance to set them right. Therefore, throughout this book, we have emphasized the vital role of our teeth in keeping us feeling and looking good!

There are several other factors that contribute to the

negative sentiment about dentistry, and from these very issues arise the apprehensions that people harbour today about dental treatment. Fortunately, rapid advances have taken place in dental science and dentistry. Coupled with this, there has been a sea change in the approach of dental healthcare providers, to the entire process of rendering treatment. These have come a long way in addressing the common concerns, as well as in turning around the entire dental experience, to a positive, pleasant one.

Let's take a closer look at all the roadblocks, and how the science of modern dentistry can overcome them and carve a smoother journey.

Expectation

Dental treatment ought to be cheaper; it's just too expensive!

Elucidation

Concerns over the cost of dental procedures are often a prime consideration in avoiding treatment. Now here's a little secret: one of the biggest reasons it becomes expensive is *delay!*

People avoid going to the dentist until the eleventh hour, postponing basic treatment options like routine checks, cleaning, or simple fillings. By procrastinating thus, one worsens the existing condition, often making it more painful—and importantly—the treatment far more expensive.

The saying: 'A stitch in time saves nine' couldn't be more apt as far as dental care is concerned! The truth of the matter is that if one gets regular checkups and prompt attention, dental care is economical. It also takes fewer visits to the clinic to fix problems that are detected early, and treatment

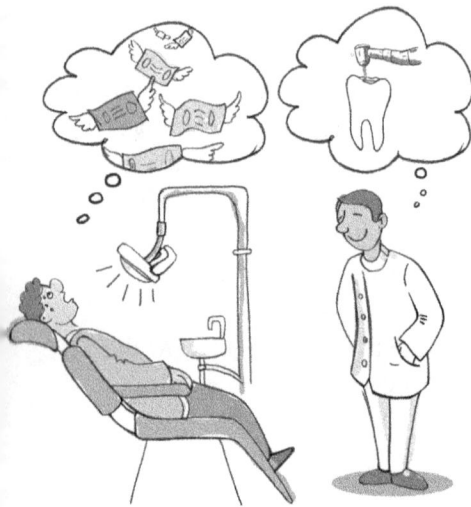

is provided with minimal discomfort.

For example, shallow cavities can be fixed with simple, inexpensive fillings. But, if the same cavity digs deep, the tooth will end up requiring extensive redressals like root canal treatment, or worse, an extraction, in case it is beyond redemption. Even after that, the operations are not over! The tooth will need replacement, and the better options for this turn out more expensive, and require more dental visits, eating up more and more of one's valuable time and resources.

Besides, the field of dentistry is very space and capital intensive, and runs with high overheads too. Dentists need to invest in fixed premises, as they cannot shuttle around town with their cumbersome machinery! The equipment itself is capital intensive; other than the dental chair, there is a wide range of essential mechanical accessories and devices in a standard dental clinic. The materials used in dentistry—specialized, high quality products—are not inexpensive. In fact, some of the composite resins for tooth fillings cost more than pure gold! The costs of outsourcing production of crowns, bridges, veneers, etc. to dental laboratories—and depending on the quality and the expertise of the technician—can cost a pretty packet. And let's not forget the salaries of staff, including receptionists, dental assistants, hygienists and housekeeping personnel! Infrastructural costs like electricity, telephones, computers and Internet, maintenance, insurance, office supplies, etc. are other basic expenses that add to the bill. Moreover, dentists also need to regularly upgrade their equipment, and their knowledge and skills.

There are hugely varying prices for the same procedure in different clinics, reflecting the cost of inputs, the location of the practice, and the skill of the practitioner. Less expensive treatments are made possible by using basic materials, simpler procedures and less experienced dentists. As a result, it is not always possible to run cost comparisons across the range of clinics.

Eventually, good quality treatment works out cheaper, as it lasts longer, and performs better. It is best to consider the outlay on dental treatment as an investment, and not as an expense!

Expectation

My treatment needs to be done quickly, with minimum visits.

Elucidation

Not too long ago, dental therapy was delivered over several episodes, like a soap opera! Procedures were lengthy, often leading to physical and mental fatigue for patients, and resulting in dropouts and incomplete treatment. 'The dentist keeps calling me repeatedly, and my treatment's just not getting over!' Statements like this were pretty commonplace, but the tide has now changed! Brace yourself for the current scenario; it can be a blink-and-miss job.

Earlier, most dentists would refer you elsewhere for getting your X-rays done. Today, digital X-rays are the norm— the dentist puts an X-ray sensor into your mouth, and at the click of a button, the image flashes *instantly* on a computer screen! No washing of films, no mess.

By and large, clinics also have their own facilities for X-ray imaging of the entire jaw—these 'panoramic' scans having gone digital too. Among the latest innovations is the cone-beam CT, which can churn out 3-D views of the jaw and skull in a trice, helping to identify early damage before it becomes apparent via conventional diagnostic techniques.

Checking for cavities has gone high-tech, with laser-based systems (like Diagnodent™) pinpointing decayed areas at the flick of a button.

Charting the condition of the gums in detail is relatively time-consuming: the dentist has to measure the gum condition around each tooth, and fill out a complex form. A new device, the Periometer™, notes the gum condition applying a computer-controlled standard force. The data obtained is stored digitally, and the docking station easily transfers it to a graph for simple reading.

Happily for both dentists and patients, many of the traditional treatments have been turned on their heads over the last few years! Improvements in technology have revolutionized the speed and efficacy of most dental procedures.

Extraction of broken teeth has become more refined, and quicker with the use of Luxators™—fine bladed instruments which help the dentist avoid lengthy dissection of gum and bone tissue to remove such teeth.

Scaling, or the cleaning of teeth, is no longer done by manual scraping. Ultrasonic scalers do the job efficiently, comfortably and many times faster.

Root canal treatment has been dramatically simplified by the use of rotary systems. These are motor-driven flexible cutting files, which can complete the cleaning and shaping of the root canals in minutes. As a result, most treatments done today are completed in a single sitting!

Operating microscopes are also making their way into dental clinics—the magnified view of the intricate structures within the tooth accelerating the dentist's work manifold.

Taking impressions of the teeth is necessary for many procedures, such as the production of crowns and bridges—a slightly messy, gooey process, which adds to treatment time. Now, with digital scanners (such as iTero™), after the necessary shaping of the tooth, the dentist scans the mouth, and the digital images are directly transferred to the dental laboratory.

Crowns and bridges are traditionally made in a laboratory using the models from tooth impressions prepared by the dentist. Several days can pass for the product to be finally fixed to the jaw. The latest technology brings 'in-office CAD-CAM', a machine that receives the digital images of your tooth as prepared by the dentist, and creates a 3-D representation of it. Based on this, the machine mills out a crown or bridge, as necessary, using a CAD-CAM technique. The whole process is over in a couple of hours!

Lasers are speeding up many aspects of dental treatment. Soft-tissue models, such as the CO_2 or diode, are more common, and are used for minor surgeries and conservative gum treatment. Argon lasers ensure rapid whitening of teeth, and also faster curing of composite fillings. For hard-tissues, an Erbium laser is amongst those that are effective in the conservative removal of tooth decay, and the shaping and contouring of bone during surgical work. Lasers work fast, ensure a bloodless field, and promote quicker healing—this obviously benefits you and your dentist both!

And there's much that has changed in the 'administrative' environment too. Intelligent scheduling, or block scheduling of appointments, helps dentists operate efficiently, also offering huge savings in time for you. A lengthy sitting is reserved for your treatment, accomplishing in one long session what would've otherwise spilled over into multiple visits. Plenty of rest intervals are factored into such marathons, to minimize strain to your jaws. Cyber-savvy clinics can make IT work for you: booking appointments over the Internet, reminders for your appointment, cellphone apps with GPS to provide precise directions, and real-time maps to help you find the clinic, etc. Some cellphone apps supplied by your dentist also educate you about dental health, furnish illustrations of your dental condition, and display your treatment plan amongst other items of information.

Expectation

My dental treatment shouldn't compromise my appearance—I need to continue going to work or party, without any inhibitions!

Elucidation

In today's demanding world, which places a premium on your appearance, dental treatment cannot afford to play spoilsport. During its course, teeth may have to be removed, or shaped down for crowns or bridges, and implants might have to be inserted. The final replacements could occasionally be delayed to accommodate healing, or final restorations wait out the fabrication period in the laboratory.

But, unfortunately, work constraints and social engagements cannot tarry! Well, entirely cognizant of these facts, dentists and their tools are now increasingly tuned towards ensuring that your face is not affected by ongoing treatment.

When prepared teeth are awaiting crowns and/or bridges, temporary mimics are made on the spot, and fixed into place with removable cements. This ensures that you don't need to walk around trying to hide your gap-toothed look, or your oddly shaped teeth.

When a dental implant is placed in the visible zone (for instance, on the front row) it is now possible to immediately place a temporary crown over it—called immediate loading—to cover the abnormality.

When a visible tooth is removed, a customized immediate partial denture can be substituted directly after the extraction. Similarly, even an immediate complete denture can be placed instantly, after removal of all the teeth. These dentures serve to preserve facial appearance and speech, and are fairly functional too!

Orthodontic treatment includes various aesthetic options as well: tooth-coloured wires and brackets, invisible aligners, wires fixed on the inner aspects of the teeth, etc. Today, with adults increasingly opting for Orthodontic therapy, these fittings are now commonplace, avoiding the embarrassment of being seen with braces at the office!

Expectation

I shouldn't catch any bug at the dentist's—the instruments used must've gone into so many mouths!

Elucidation

We are all justifiably concerned about hygiene at any establishment seeing a great deal of human traffic, be it a restaurant or a restroom!

Dentistry falls under the category of surgical treatment, due to which dental clinics are akin to minor operation theatres. Protocols for maintaining strict hygiene are built into the routine.

Any instrument used in the mouth is either disposed of, or undergoes sterilization in a prescribed manner, usually through autoclaving—steam sterilization under high pressure. Even the drills need to be autoclaved, due to which operatories have an inventory of multiple drills, to suffice for a day's routine. Sterilization using boiling water is now obsolete, as it falls short of the standard. Indeed, some instruments are sterilized by using powerful chemical solutions, such as glutaraldehyde. Even the impressions sent to the dental laboratory are disinfected before use!

Sterile disposable gloves, face-masks, face shields, gowns, suction machine tips, etc. are used by default to protect against infection, and prevent any cross contamination between patients. Syringes, needles and single-dose units of local anaesthetics are all used strictly as disposables.

All surfaces of objects in the dental operatory touched by operators during treatment, are either covered with disposable barrier films, or disinfected chemically after each use. Operatory floors and other fixed surfaces are sanitized regularly throughout the day.

Dentists incorporate these measures as part of their SOP (standard operating procedures). If you are concerned about catching infections, or about the sterilization and hygiene practices, please discuss it with your dentist. You will realize that you can sit back and relax—the only thing you may catch is an infectious smile!

Expectation

I don't want to feel embarrassed—my teeth are a mess, and the dentist's going to yell!

Elucidation

Many of us procrastinate when it comes to seeking timely attention for our teeth. We allow deposits to build up, teeth to get stained, and gums to swell up. We ignore smaller cavities, which only get larger. Some teeth actually break away, leaving only the roots behind. We develop halitosis, and become self-conscious about the state of our teeth. We even try to smile without showing them! Naturally, we are a bit ashamed about all this, and when it's time to see the dentist, we shy away—feeling like a mortified child showing a poor report card to the parent!

Take heart—dentists have spent a better part of their lives looking at bad teeth! They may certainly opine that you could've come in earlier, but will get down to the business of planning your treatment without sermonizing. Who better than a dentist to understand your tendency to avoid dental therapy? They are professionals offering a service, and no longer fancy delivering lectures from a high moral ground—they know that this can be counterproductive, forcing you to again withdraw into your shell and turn away.

Dentists are more focused on how to fix your problem, and get your teeth back on track quickly. It is never too late to seek help—broken teeth can be mended, seemingly hopeless teeth saved, and the really bad ones removed, only to be replaced by lifelike substitutes.

The issue with neglected teeth is that they end up needing more complex treatment, and require a larger number of sittings. If you are abashed by the way your teeth look, you can ask your dentist to solve that issue first—thereafter, with your increased confidence you are more likely to follow through on the rest of the treatment!

And do remember, for every dentist who pontificates or berates you for having neglected your teeth, you can find a dozen who are empathetic, and appreciative of the fact that you have sought their help to fix them!

Expectation

Dentists shouldn't pretend to be doctors! They are akin to overeducated technicians.

Elucidation

Dentistry has had very shadowy beginnings shrouded in the mists of time it is true. Dental techniques were violent, painful, and often performed by unqualified people. In fact, there was a phase when barbers rendered this treatment! Sadly, this unsavoury history has managed to allow its dubious legacy to filter down into our uber-modern world.

Many people still harbour a very poor image of dentists, considering them mere 'tooth-pullers' who enjoy inflicting pain. They are often seen as second-class practitioners, who weren't bright enough to qualify as 'real' doctors. As a result, there is a tendency to avoid seeking professional help for dental problems, and even when dentists are consulted their advice is viewed with suspicion!

Here are a few facts about contemporary dental professionals to help put matters into perspective. Dentists train for a minimum of five years during their undergraduate course. Specialization takes up another three years. That's eight years of education—as much as any other medical specialist! During their training, they learn every single aspect of the curriculum followed by medical students AND receive specialized training in dentistry too, from the word go!

Imagine the skill you would require to operate inside a tiny, dark, wet structure, using ultra-high speed drills. To add to the excitement, a tongue snakes about, blood and fluids obscure your vision, and for half of the area you need a mirror to be able to view your workings! If you recognize this structure as the mouth, you will appreciate the amazing hand-eye coordination, and high level of manual dexterity, that dentists possess!

Most dental procedures are performed on fully conscious patients, who are often apprehensive. Dentists still measure up to the challenge of maintaining accurate focus and precise control so as to work safely, and to deliver results.

The dentist is a one-man team, performing a wide range of procedures! Dentists must administer anaesthesia, do their own X-rays and reporting, perform surgeries including plastic surgery and use drugs to treat mouth ailments. They use lasers, detect cancers, help diagnose diabetes and stress and also counsel their patients. And, oh yes, they fill and pull out teeth as well!

Let's take a sneak peek at some of the cutting edge developments currently coming out of dental research labs—expectations that are entering the realm of reality:

- Growing new teeth in a lab, from stem cells: Don't worry if you lose your tooth, a new one can be formed from your own stem cells in replacement.
- Germ warfare: Genetically modified bacteria are being used to target the cavity-causing germs in the mouth. Don't throw away your toothbrush just yet, but soon, you could possibly use a mouth rinse containing these good critters to banish cavities!
- Nanodentistry: This is the new kid in the block! 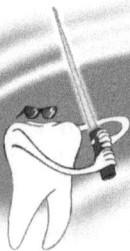 Microscopic robots, called nanorobots, can be used to keep the mouth clean by eliminating bacteria. They can numb specific teeth, or desensitize exposed dentin. Tooth alignments could be corrected in minutes by using nanorobots to tweak the periodontal ligament and jawbone! And, they can also be programmed to selectively kill cancer cells.
- Dentists are your partners in caring for your oral health. They lend the professional edge in preserving and maintaining your teeth for a lifetime. Healthy teeth translate into good overall wellbeing, and pave the way for a great quality of life.

Keep smiling!

Glossary of Dental Specialists

The evolution of dentistry into a modern, advanced branch of medical science was spurred by intensive study and in-depth research. This has led to the creation of several specialities in this already specialized field. Most dentists practice as general dental practitioners, offering a vast spectrum of treatment procedures. However, some challenging situations are better tackled by specialists. Here's a list:

Oral and maxillofacial surgeons focus on surgical treatment within the mouth and pertaining to the jaws, such as surgical removal of impacted teeth, cysts and tumours, and surgeries for correcting jaw defects.

Periodontists, also known as gum specialists, deal with putting the gums back on track using a combination of surgical and non-surgical treatment.

Orthodontists are familiar dental specialists working on realigning crooked teeth using various forms of braces.

Paedodontists focus on dental treatment for kids and are trained to render preventive as well as corrective treatment for children up to the age of twelve.

Prosthodontists specialize in all forms of tooth replacement—dentures, bridges, implants, as well as special devices for those who have deformities caused by cleft palate, cancer surgery, etc.

Oral pathologists devote their skills to the microscopic study of tumours, growths and other lesions in the mouth.

Endodontists specialize in the intricacies of root canal treatment in its various forms, including surgical treatment of the roots.

Oral and maxillofacial radiologists study the teeth and jaws using X-rays, scans, etc.

Dental public health specialists focus on oral and dental health for the community as a whole through education, awareness, programmes for the prevention of disease, etc.

Apart from these nine specialities, recognized even by the American Dental Association, other specialities are emerging too—such as *cosmetic dentistry*, which focuses on enhancing the beauty of your smile, and *dental implantology*, devoted to the science of dental implants.

Acknowledgements

First and foremost, I would like to thank my most adorable parents, Anasuya and Balachandran Menon for believing that their daughter is the best—for educating me and always providing for me despite all the hardships they endured. All my gratitude to my dearest brother, Suraj who patted me on the back, wiped my tears or chided me, as the occasion demanded.

I would like to thank my extended family—Babumama and Paicheriamma, Sujit, Dinesh, Sushma, Deepti, Radhika, Sheela, Ponnaellacha, the late Hariellayachcha, Leela and Devi Cheriamma and Acchayamma for their unflinching love and admiration for me, the acknowledged family brat.

I am eternally grateful to my teachers, Rammamurthy Sir, Mrs Lee and Mrs Raman for guiding me early in my school days in Atomic Energy Secondary School and Junior College. It goes without saying I would not be a practising dentist if not for amazing teachers like Dr Hemant Dhusia and the late Dr Mrs Annie John from my alma mater, Government Dental College and Hospital, Mumbai.

I am grateful to all my patients over the last twenty-five years, who have helped me become not only a sincere dentist but also a better human being. I value each and every one for treating me as a granddaughter, daughter, sister, friend or aunt. I would like to specifically thank all the toddlers and young children who have trusted me blindly with their treatment and have left the clinic, planting a kiss on my cheeks. (A father's offer to do the same was politely declined, of course.) I am grateful to my dental assistants, Anita, Dhanu, Sumati, and receptionists, Gayatri and Ayesha without whose hard work and sincerity we would never be able to manage our strict schedule and wonderful practice for decades. I must also thank my dental laboratory technicians who have over the years helped create the wonderful smiles of my patients.

I am grateful to all my friends, old and new, who have encouraged, pampered and loved me unconditionally over the years.

I know it is clichéd but I have to thank my loving pets, Frisky, Toughie, Chickoo, Sweetie, Tigeroos, Patchy, Kunjee, GT, Gooblish, Bouncy, Goondoos, Blackie and Paplu who have been an important part of my life, and have never judged me, but only showered their love on me.

Last but definitely not the least, I would like to thank Subbu for the wondrous togetherness we have shared since June 1992.

—Dr Sarita Subramaniam

As a child, I was told that I was destined to lead a hand-to-mouth existence, so I chose to be a dentist!

I am thankful to my parents for their unstinting support and encouragement—not only by giving me a professional education but also by helping me set up a dental practice. I also wish to acknowledge the role of my brother, Dr P.V. Vaidyanathan in leading me towards dentistry.

I am grateful to Dr K.S. Banga for being a brother, friend, guide and philosopher; my classmates, Drs Rajesh Menon, Sharukh Khajotia, Joydeep Ghosh, Arun Subramaniam, Satshil Sabnis, Prakash Advani and Sanjay Bhagalia for being my safety net in the early years; Dr A. Kumaraswamy for granting me my first taste of private practice and for being a valuable mentor; and all my wonderful teachers at the Nair Hospital Dental College (from 1984 to 1990) who selflessly shared their knowledge and held my hand, guiding me through a tough and challenging course. I must thank my good friend, Dr Udatta Kher for pushing me into the world of dental implants; my innumerable colleagues for sharing their experiences and wisdom over the years; Suresh, Sunitha and Sanju for blindly trusting my abilities; and my oldest friend, Vinay Bose for being my first patient!

I would like to acknowledge the invaluable role played by my patients through the years—their respect and their faith in me has only spurred me on to learn more and become a better dentist.

And last, but not the least, to my 'partner in crime', Sarita for playing the roles of wife, friend, colleague, advisor, sounding board and sympathizer to perfection!

Both of us would also like to place on record our appreciation for Anita Sundareswaran—a hugely talented artist and designer—for creating the wonderful illustrations that enliven the chapters. We would also like to thank Maithili Doshi Aphale from Rupa for the cover design.

We are indebted to Rupa Publications for reposing faith in this book, and the editor, Dharini Bhaskar for greatly adding value to the manuscript. Finally, we must thank Priya Doraswamy of Lotus Lane, our literary agent, for not only goading us into writing the book, but for being with us through the entire journey!

—Dr P.V. Subramaniam

www.ingramcontent.com/pod-product-compliance
Lightning Source LLC
Chambersburg PA
CBHW020607270326
41927CB00005B/213